CKD STA
TYPE 2 COOKBOOK FOR BEGINNERS

MW01169825

Complete guide to Healthy low in sodium, phosphorus and potassium kidney-friendly and diabetes diet recipes.

Olivia Endwell

Copyright Statement:

Disclaimer:

The information provided in this book is for educational and informational purposes only. It is not intended as a substitute for professional medical advice, diagnosis, or treatment. Always seek the advice of your physician or other qualified health provider with any questions you may have regarding a medical condition. Never disregard professional medical advice or delay in seeking it because of something you have read in this book.

The author and publisher disclaim any liability arising directly or indirectly from the use of this book. The information provided is based on the author's best knowledge at the time of writing and is subject to change. The author and publisher do not guarantee the accuracy, completeness, or timeliness of the information presented in this book.

Individual results may vary, and the success of any dietary or lifestyle change depends on various factors, including but not limited to individual commitment and adherence. Before making significant changes to your diet or lifestyle, consult with a qualified healthcare professional.

The views and opinions expressed in this book are those of the author and do not necessarily reflect the official policy or position of any other agency, organization, employer, or company.

TABLE OF CONTENTS

INTRODUCTION

Welcome to a journey of nourishment, well-being, and empowerment! If you've found your way to this cookbook, chances are you or someone close to you is grappling with the complex interplay of Chronic Kidney Disease (CKD) Stage 3 and Type 2 Diabetes. Navigating the landscape of these health challenges can feel like an uphill climb, filled with uncertainties and questions about where to start. We get it – the journey is personal, and we're here to guide you through it.

Before we delve into the recipes that will not only satisfy your taste buds but also align with your health goals, let's take a moment to understand what CKD Stage 3 and Diabetes Type 2 really mean. Chronic Kidney Disease, often referred to as CKD, is a condition where your kidneys aren't functioning at their best. When it reaches Stage 3, it signifies a moderate decrease in kidney function. Meanwhile, Type 2 Diabetes, a condition characterized by insulin resistance, adds another layer of complexity. These two conditions often go hand in hand, influencing each other in ways that require a thoughtful and tailored approach to management.

We acknowledge the daily challenges you face – the monitoring, the medications, the dietary restrictions. It's not just about managing one condition; it's about finding the delicate balance that accommodates both, allowing you to live a full and vibrant life. In this cookbook, we aim to provide you with practical insights, delicious recipes, and a sense of control over your culinary choices.

Now, let's talk about the cornerstone of your journey – nutrition. In managing CKD Stage 3 and Type 2 Diabetes, what you eat becomes more than just fuel; it's a crucial component of your overall well-being. Nutrition plays a pivotal role in supporting kidney function, regulating blood sugar levels, and promoting a healthy lifestyle. However, the challenge lies in finding a balance that caters to the specific needs of both conditions.

Traditional cookbooks might not cut it when you're dealing with this intricate tapestry of health concerns. That's why this cookbook is more than a collection of recipes – it's your culinary companion on this journey. We recognize that your diet isn't just about sustenance; it's a tool for managing your health. Our goal is to empower you with knowledge about nutrient-rich ingredients, portion control, and mindful eating, all woven into the fabric of flavorsome dishes that bring joy to your table.

So, how can this cookbook make a difference in your life? It's not about reinventing the wheel but rather offering you a roadmap tailored to your unique needs. Here's how:

Practical Guidance: We understand that implementing dietary changes can be overwhelming. That's why we've crafted this cookbook with simplicity in mind. You'll find easy-to-follow recipes, each with a focus on accessible ingredients and straightforward instructions. No complex culinary acrobatics – just good food that supports your health.

Variety and Flavor: Healthy eating should never equate to bland or monotonous meals. Our recipes celebrate the diversity of flavors, textures, and cuisines, ensuring that your journey towards better health is as delightful as it is nutritious. From breakfast to dinner and everything in between, you'll discover a spectrum of tastes that cater to your preferences.

Empowering Choices: This cookbook isn't about dictating what you should eat; it's about providing you with the tools to make informed and empowering choices. We offer insights into ingredient substitutions, meal planning, and smart choices when dining out. Consider it your go-to resource for crafting meals that align with your health objectives.

As you embark on this culinary exploration, remember that you're not alone. Many individuals face similar challenges, and our aim is to foster a sense of community and support through the pages of this cookbook. Together, we can turn the seemingly intricate dance of managing CKD Stage 3 and Type 2 Diabetes into a harmonious and enjoyable journey.

So, grab your apron, preheat the oven, and let's embark on this flavorful adventure towards a healthier, happier you.

BASICS OF CKD STAGE 3 AND DIABETES TYPE 2

Chronic Kidney Disease (CKD) Stage 3 and Type 2 Diabetes are formidable health challenges that, when combined, create a complex interplay requiring careful consideration and management. In this section, we'll delve into the foundational knowledge essential for navigating these conditions effectively.

Overview of CKD Stage 3

CKD is a progressive condition where the kidneys, vital organs responsible for filtering waste and excess fluids from the blood, gradually lose their function over time. In Stage 3, the disease advances beyond the early stages, indicating a moderate decline in kidney function. This is a critical juncture where proactive measures become pivotal in slowing the progression of the disease.

The hallmark of Stage 3 CKD is a glomerular filtration rate (GFR) between 30 and 59 milliliters per minute, reflecting a reduced ability of the kidneys to filter blood effectively. Symptoms might not be overt at this stage, making regular monitoring and early intervention crucial. Individuals with Stage 3 CKD may experience increased blood pressure, changes in urine output, and potential imbalances in electrolytes.

Understanding the nuances of Stage 3 CKD involves recognizing its potential causes, such as diabetes, hypertension, or other underlying conditions. Additionally, grasping the significance of regular check-ups, blood tests, and adherence to prescribed medications is key to managing CKD effectively. Knowledge is the first line of defense, empowering individuals to actively participate in their health journey.

Understanding Diabetes Type 2

Type 2 Diabetes, a metabolic disorder, is characterized by insulin resistance, where the body's cells become less responsive to insulin, the hormone responsible for regulating blood sugar levels. This insulin resistance, coupled with inadequate insulin production, leads to elevated blood glucose levels. Unlike Type 1 Diabetes, which is an autoimmune condition where the body doesn't produce insulin at all, Type 2 Diabetes often develops later in life and is closely tied to lifestyle factors.

Understanding the intricacies of Type 2 Diabetes involves recognizing the role of insulin in glucose metabolism. When cells resist insulin, glucose remains in the bloodstream, causing hyperglycemia. This condition, if left unmanaged, can lead to a range of complications, including cardiovascular issues, nerve damage, and kidney problems.

Lifestyle factors, including diet, exercise, and genetics, play a significant role in the development and progression of Type 2 Diabetes. Awareness of risk factors, such as obesity, sedentary lifestyle, and a family history of diabetes, empowers individuals to make informed choices for prevention and management. Regular monitoring of blood sugar levels, adopting a balanced diet, and engaging in physical activity are fundamental components of diabetes care.

Interconnection between CKD and Diabetes

The intricate dance between CKD Stage 3 and Type 2 Diabetes is a complex interconnection that amplifies the challenges faced by individuals dealing with both conditions simultaneously. Diabetes is a leading cause of CKD, and when these two conditions coexist, they create a synergistic impact, each influencing the progression and management of the other.

The relationship between CKD and Diabetes is bidirectional. Diabetes can contribute to the development and progression of CKD by damaging the blood vessels in the kidneys and impairing their ability to function properly. On the other hand, CKD can exacerbate diabetes by causing insulin resistance, leading to poorer blood sugar control.

Understanding this interconnection is paramount for effective management. Individuals with both CKD Stage 3 and Type 2 Diabetes require a holistic approach that addresses the unique challenges posed by each condition while recognizing their shared impact. Lifestyle modifications, including dietary changes, exercise, and medication adherence, become crucial elements in breaking the cycle of mutual influence between CKD and Diabetes.

Managing these conditions requires a comprehensive strategy that considers the implications of one on the other. For instance, controlling blood sugar levels becomes not only a diabetes management goal but also a measure to preserve kidney function. Likewise, interventions to slow the progression of CKD can positively impact diabetes control.

Moreover, medications used to manage diabetes may need adjustments to accommodate kidney function, as impaired kidneys may affect the clearance of certain drugs from the body. Collaborative care between healthcare providers specializing in diabetes and nephrology is essential to ensure a cohesive and effective management plan.

In essence, the interconnection between CKD Stage 3 and Type 2 Diabetes underscores the need for a nuanced and integrated approach to healthcare. It emphasizes the importance of a healthcare team that works together, taking into account the unique challenges presented by these coexisting conditions. This collaborative effort extends beyond the clinic or hospital, involving individuals in actively managing their health through informed decision-making and lifestyle choices.

DIETARY GUIDELINES FOR CKD AND DIABETES

Navigating the dietary landscape when facing both Chronic Kidney Disease (CKD) and Type 2 Diabetes requires a tailored and thoughtful approach. This section aims to elucidate the essential dietary guidelines that form the cornerstone of managing these coexisting conditions.

General Dietary Recommendations

In the realm of CKD and Diabetes, general dietary recommendations are fundamental guidelines that lay the groundwork for a health-supportive eating plan. These recommendations are not one-size-fits-all but serve as a flexible framework to guide individuals in making informed and health-conscious choices.

First and foremost, a balanced and nutritious diet is crucial. This includes a variety of fruits, vegetables, whole grains, lean proteins, and healthy fats. The emphasis on diversity ensures a broad spectrum of essential nutrients, promoting overall health and well-being.

When crafting a meal plan, attention to portion control is paramount. Monitoring portion sizes helps regulate calorie intake, supporting weight management – a crucial aspect for individuals with Type 2 Diabetes. Additionally, it aids in controlling phosphorus and potassium levels, essential considerations for those with CKD.

8

Limiting sodium intake is another key recommendation. Excessive sodium can contribute to elevated blood pressure, a risk factor for both CKD and Diabetes. Choosing fresh, whole foods and minimizing the use of processed or pre-packaged items can significantly reduce sodium intake.

Hydration is often underestimated but holds significant importance. Maintaining adequate fluid intake helps support kidney function and can aid in controlling blood sugar levels. However, fluid intake may need to be adjusted based on individual health status and CKD stage, highlighting the need for personalized dietary recommendations.

Understanding and managing carbohydrate intake is crucial for individuals with Diabetes. Choosing complex carbohydrates with a low glycemic index helps regulate blood sugar levels. Fiber-rich foods, such as whole grains and legumes, contribute to sustained energy and digestive health.

In essence, these general dietary recommendations create a solid foundation for individuals managing CKD and Diabetes. They promote a holistic and balanced approach to nutrition, considering the unique needs and challenges presented by both conditions.

Importance of Monitoring Nutrient Intake

Monitoring nutrient intake goes beyond merely counting calories; it involves a nuanced understanding of the impact of specific nutrients on both CKD and Diabetes. This level of awareness becomes particularly vital in managing these conditions where dietary choices directly influence health outcomes.

For individuals with CKD, closely monitoring protein intake is a key consideration. While protein is essential for overall health, excessive protein consumption can strain the kidneys. This is especially relevant in the context of Diabetes, where kidney function may already be compromised. A dietitian can provide personalized recommendations to strike the right balance between maintaining adequate protein levels for bodily functions and preventing excess load on the kidneys.

Phosphorus and potassium are minerals that require vigilant oversight in CKD. Imbalances can arise due to reduced kidney function, leading to complications. Foods high in phosphorus, such as dairy products and nuts, should be moderated, and potassium-rich foods, like bananas and oranges, may need careful management. Monitoring these minerals supports kidney health and prevents further complications.

For individuals with Diabetes, a crucial nutrient to monitor is carbohydrates. Carbohydrate counting is a valuable tool in managing blood sugar levels. Understanding the carbohydrate content of foods empowers individuals to make informed choices and better control their diabetes.

Furthermore, attention to dietary fats is essential. Healthy fats, such as those found in avocados and olive oil, can be beneficial. However, moderation is key, as excessive fat intake can contribute to weight gain, impacting both blood sugar control and overall health.

Vitamins and minerals, including vitamin D and calcium, also warrant attention. Reduced kidney function can affect the body's ability to activate vitamin D, impacting bone health. Adequate calcium intake, while considering phosphorus levels, is crucial to maintain bone density.

In essence, monitoring nutrient intake involves a meticulous examination of the nutritional content of foods and its potential impact on kidney function and blood sugar control. This level of awareness allows individuals to make informed choices that align with their health goals, providing a proactive and personalized approach to dietary management.

Special Considerations for CKD and Diabetes

The amalgamation of CKD and Diabetes necessitates special considerations that go beyond general dietary guidelines. These considerations acknowledge the unique challenges posed by each condition and aim to create a tailored approach to dietary management.

One of the primary considerations is the need for individualized meal plans. CKD and Diabetes manifest differently in each person, and the impact of diet can vary widely. Collaborating with a registered dietitian becomes imperative to create a plan that addresses specific health needs, considering factors such as CKD stage, medications, and personal preferences.

Limiting phosphorus and potassium becomes more pronounced in this context. Foods that are typically considered healthy may need to be moderated or substituted. For example, high-potassium fruits may need to be replaced with lower-potassium alternatives, and phosphorus-containing additives may require scrutiny on food labels.

Fluid restriction is a common recommendation for those with advanced CKD, particularly in later stages. While staying adequately hydrated is crucial, strict fluid control may be necessary to prevent complications like fluid retention. This delicate balance requires collaboration with healthcare providers and dietitians to tailor recommendations to individual needs.

Individuals with Diabetes and CKD also face the challenge of managing blood sugar levels while being mindful of their kidney health. This involves strategic meal planning that considers both carbohydrate content and the impact on kidney function. Regular monitoring of blood sugar levels and adjustments to the meal plan based on these readings become integral components of diabetes management in this context.

Sodium restriction, already emphasized in general dietary recommendations, takes on additional significance in the presence of CKD. Managing blood pressure is a key goal, and sodium reduction plays a pivotal role. Choosing fresh, unprocessed foods and minimizing the use of salt in cooking become essential practices.

In summary, special considerations for CKD and Diabetes involve a highly personalized approach to dietary management. Collaboration with healthcare professionals, especially dietitians, is paramount to creating a plan that not only supports overall health but also addresses the intricacies of these coexisting conditions. This tailored approach acknowledges the diverse nature of CKD and Diabetes and empowers individuals to take an active role in managing their health through informed dietary choices.

CKD AND DIABETES-FRIENDLY INGREDIENTS

When it comes to managing the intricate balance of Chronic Kidney Disease (CKD) and Type 2 Diabetes, the choice of ingredients becomes paramount. This section unravels the realm of CKD and diabetes-friendly ingredients, focusing on low-potassium and low-phosphorus options, low-glycemic index foods, and the selection of healthy fats and proteins.

Low-Potassium and Low-Phosphorus Options

For individuals navigating the confluence of CKD and Diabetes, keeping a watchful eye on potassium and phosphorus levels in their diet is crucial. Elevated potassium levels, known as hyperkalemia, can pose risks for those with compromised kidney function. Similarly, excess phosphorus can contribute to complications, particularly in the context of CKD. Therefore, incorporating low-potassium and low-phosphorus options becomes a strategic approach to support overall health.

Low-Potassium Options:

Fruits and vegetables are often rich in potassium, but not all are created equal. Opting for low-potassium choices can include berries (such as strawberries and blueberries), apples, and cauliflower. These alternatives provide essential vitamins and minerals without burdening the kidneys with excessive potassium.

When it comes to proteins, selecting lean cuts of meat, poultry, or fish can help control potassium intake. Additionally, cooking methods like boiling and leaching can further reduce potassium content, making these proteins kidney-friendly choices.

Low-Phosphorus Options:

Phosphorus is prevalent in many foods, particularly processed and packaged items. Navigating towards low-phosphorus alternatives involves choosing whole, fresh foods. Grains like rice and oats, as well as fresh fruits and vegetables, are generally lower in phosphorus. Dairy substitutes, such as almond or rice milk, can be considered to manage phosphorus intake.

In the realm of proteins, eggs, poultry, and certain cuts of pork can be lower in phosphorus. Plant-based protein sources like tofu and legumes are also viable options. However, portion control remains essential, as even low-phosphorus foods can contribute to elevated levels when consumed excessively.

Low-Glycemic Index Foods

Managing blood sugar levels is a primary concern for individuals with Type 2 Diabetes, and the glycemic index (GI) provides valuable insight into how different foods affect blood glucose levels. Choosing low-GI foods is a strategic approach to promote stable blood sugar control, aligning with the objectives of diabetes management.

Low-GI Options:

Whole grains, such as quinoa and barley, are excellent choices for individuals with CKD and Diabetes. These grains release glucose gradually, preventing sudden spikes in blood sugar. Non-starchy vegetables, like leafy greens and broccoli, are also low on the glycemic index, providing essential nutrients without compromising blood sugar control.

Legumes, such as lentils and chickpeas, offer a double benefit by providing plant-based protein along with a low-GI profile. Fruits like berries and cherries are flavorful additions that score low on the glycemic index, making them suitable for those managing diabetes.

Incorporating these low-GI foods into daily meals contributes not only to stable blood sugar levels but also aligns with the dietary guidelines for CKD, emphasizing whole, nutrient-dense choices.

Healthy Fats and Proteins

Dietary fats and proteins are integral components of a balanced diet, but when managing CKD and Diabetes, the emphasis shifts to selecting healthy options that support overall health without overburdening compromised kidneys or exacerbating diabetes.

Healthy Fats:

In the context of CKD and Diabetes, healthy fats take center stage. Opting for monounsaturated and polyunsaturated fats can positively impact heart health, a critical consideration for those with diabetes. Olive oil, avocados, and nuts are excellent sources of monounsaturated fats, providing flavorful additions to meals without compromising health.

Omega-3 fatty acids, found in fatty fish like salmon and mackerel, contribute to heart health and may have anti-inflammatory effects, offering additional benefits for individuals managing both CKD and Diabetes. Flaxseeds and chia seeds are plant-based sources of omega-3s, catering to various dietary preferences.

Healthy Proteins:

When it comes to proteins, quality matters more than quantity. For individuals with CKD, focusing on high-quality, lean protein sources becomes essential. Fish, poultry, and plant-based proteins like tofu and legumes offer protein without excessive phosphorus, supporting kidney health.

In the realm of diabetes management, incorporating proteins that do not contribute to rapid blood sugar spikes is crucial. Lean cuts of meat, eggs, and plant-based proteins are suitable choices. Additionally, the combination of protein and healthy fats can contribute to a sense of satiety, supporting weight management – a key aspect for individuals with diabetes.

In essence, the selection of healthy fats and proteins for individuals managing CKD and Diabetes involves a thoughtful consideration of the impact on both conditions. It's about striking a balance that supports kidney health, blood sugar control, and overall well-being.

BUILDING A CKD AND DIABETES-FRIENDLY KITCHEN

Creating a kitchen that supports the management of Chronic Kidney Disease (CKD) and Type 2 Diabetes involves more than just preparing meals. It's about strategically setting up your culinary space to align with the unique dietary needs of these conditions. This section explores the essential elements of building a CKD and Diabetes-friendly kitchen, focusing on stocking your pantry, essential kitchen tools, and practical meal planning tips.

Stocking Your Pantry

A well-stocked pantry is the foundation of a CKD and Diabetes-friendly kitchen. It not only streamlines meal preparation but also ensures that you have a variety of health-supportive ingredients at your fingertips. Here's a guide to stocking your pantry with items tailored to the needs of CKD and Diabetes:

1. Low-Potassium and Low-Phosphorus Staples:

- Grains: Opt for low-phosphorus grains like rice, quinoa, and couscous. These serve as versatile bases for meals without contributing to elevated phosphorus levels.

- Pasta: Choose whole-grain pasta as a fiber-rich alternative, contributing to stable blood sugar levels and supporting overall health.

2. Canned Goods with Caution:

- Beans: Canned beans are convenient, but be mindful of sodium content. Rinse canned beans thoroughly to reduce sodium levels before use.

- Tomatoes: Canned tomatoes and tomato products are versatile, but choose low-sodium options to manage sodium intake.

3. Healthy Fats:

- Oils: Stock up on heart-healthy oils like olive oil for cooking and dressing. These provide essential fats without compromising kidney or diabetes health.

- Nuts and Seeds: Choose unsalted varieties for snacks or adding a crunch to salads. They contribute healthy fats and essential nutrients.

4. Low-Glycemic Index Sweeteners:

- Stevia or Monk Fruit: Opt for natural, low-GI sweeteners for occasional use in recipes or beverages. These alternatives can help manage blood sugar levels.

5. Herbs and Spices:

- Diversify your flavor palette with a variety of herbs and spices. Fresh or dried, these add depth to your dishes without relying on excessive salt.

6. Low-Sodium Broths and Bouillons:

- Use low-sodium broths as a base for soups and stews. These add flavor without contributing to elevated blood pressure.

Building a CKD and Diabetes-friendly pantry is about making thoughtful choices that align with the nutritional needs of both conditions. Regularly check labels for sodium and phosphorus content, and aim for whole, unprocessed options whenever possible.

Essential Kitchen Tools

Equipping your kitchen with the right tools can streamline meal preparation and make the process more enjoyable. Consider the following essential kitchen tools for a CKD and Diabetes-friendly culinary space:

1. Food Scale:

- A food scale is invaluable for portion control, especially when managing protein intake. It helps ensure that you stay within recommended limits without the guesswork.

2. Cutting Boards and Quality Knives:

- Invest in high-quality cutting boards and sharp knives. These make chopping fruits, vegetables, and proteins more efficient, contributing to an enjoyable cooking experience.

3. Non-Stick Cookware:

- Non-stick pans require less oil for cooking, promoting heart health. They also simplify clean-up, making them a practical choice for everyday use.

4. Steamer Basket:

- Steaming is a gentle cooking method that helps retain nutrients in vegetables and proteins. A steamer basket is a versatile tool for preparing kidney and diabetes-friendly meals.

5. Slow Cooker:

- A slow cooker is a time-saving and convenient tool. It allows for the preparation of flavorful, nutrient-rich meals with minimal effort. Ideal for busy days.

6. Blender or Food Processor:

- These appliances are versatile for creating smoothies, soups, and purees. They are particularly useful when incorporating fruits and vegetables into your diet.

7. Instant-Read Thermometer:

- Ensure the proper cooking of proteins with an instant-read thermometer. This helps avoid overcooking or undercooking, providing optimal taste and texture.

8. Measuring Cups and Spoons:

- Precision matters in managing both CKD and Diabetes. Accurate measuring cups and spoons are essential for portion control and following recipes closely.

9. Herb and Spice Grinder:

- Freshly ground herbs and spices enhance flavor without the need for excess salt. A grinder allows you to incorporate a variety of seasonings into your meals.

Investing in quality kitchen tools not only enhances your cooking experience but also facilitates the preparation of kidney and diabetes-friendly meals. These tools contribute to efficient meal planning and execution, making it easier to adhere to dietary guidelines.

Meal Planning Tips

Efficient meal planning is a cornerstone of successfully managing CKD and Diabetes. It involves thoughtful consideration of nutritional requirements, portion control, and variety. Here are practical meal planning tips to guide you:

1. Collaborate with a Dietitian:

- Work with a registered dietitian to create a personalized meal plan. Their expertise ensures that your dietary choices align with the specific needs of CKD and Diabetes.

2. Prioritize Nutrient-Dense Foods:

- Focus on nutrient-dense foods that offer essential vitamins and minerals. These include fresh fruits, vegetables, lean proteins, and whole grains.

3. Monitor Portion Sizes:

- Be mindful of portion sizes to avoid overconsumption of nutrients that may be problematic for CKD or Diabetes. Use measuring tools to maintain precision.

4. Include a Variety of Colors:

- A vibrant plate often signifies a well-balanced meal. Incorporate a variety of colorful fruits and vegetables to ensure a diverse range of nutrients.

5. Plan for Leftovers:

- Prepare larger batches of CKD and Diabetes-friendly recipes to have leftovers for subsequent meals. This minimizes cooking time and ensures consistency in your dietary choices.

6. Rotate Protein Sources:

- Vary protein sources to provide a spectrum of essential amino acids. This approach not only enhances flavor but also contributes to overall nutritional balance.

7. Experiment with Flavors:

- Use herbs, spices, and low-sodium seasonings to add depth and complexity to your meals. Experimenting with flavors keeps your palate engaged and encourages adherence to your dietary plan.

8. Stay Hydrated:

- Adequate hydration is essential for kidney health. Incorporate water, herbal teas, and other low-calorie beverages into your daily routine.

9. Schedule Regular Meals and Snacks:

- Establish a routine with regular meal and snack times. This helps stabilize blood sugar levels and ensures a consistent intake of nutrients throughout the day.

10. Keep a Food Journal:

- Tracking your meals can provide valuable insights into your dietary habits. A food journal can help you identify patterns, track nutrient intake, and make informed adjustments.

Successful meal planning for CKD and Diabetes is a dynamic process that adapts to individual needs and preferences. It involves a blend of nutritional knowledge, practicality, and culinary creativity to make the journey enjoyable and sustainable.

SNACK RECIPES

1. Avocado and Tomato Bruschetta

Prep Time: 10 minutes

Cooking Time: 5 minutes

Serving Size: 2 slices per serving

Ingredients:

- 1 ripe avocado, diced

- 1 cup cherry tomatoes, diced

- 2 cloves garlic, minced

- 2 tablespoons red onion, finely chopped

- 1 tablespoon fresh basil, chopped

- 1 tablespoon olive oil

- Salt and pepper to taste

- Whole grain baguette, sliced

Instructions:

1. In a bowl, combine diced avocado, cherry tomatoes, garlic, red onion, and fresh basil.

2. Drizzle olive oil over the mixture and season with salt and pepper. Gently toss to combine.

26

3. Toast the whole grain baguette slices until golden brown.

4. Spoon the avocado and tomato mixture onto the toasted baguette slices.

5. Serve immediately and enjoy this nutrient-rich, diabetic-friendly snack.

Nutritional Information (per serving):

- Calories: 150

- Protein: 2g

- Carbohydrates: 15g

- Fiber: 4g

- Fat: 10g

- Potassium: 250mg

- Phosphorus: 60mg

2. Greek Yogurt Parfait with Berries

Prep Time: 5 minutes

Cooking Time: 0 minutes

Serving Size: 1 serving

Ingredients:

- 1/2 cup Greek yogurt (unsweetened)

- 1/4 cup blueberries

- 1/4 cup strawberries, sliced

- 1 tablespoon almonds, chopped

- 1 teaspoon honey (optional)

Instructions:

1. In a glass or bowl, layer Greek yogurt at the bottom.

2. Add a layer of blueberries and then a layer of sliced strawberries.

3. Sprinkle chopped almonds on top for added crunch.

4. Optionally, drizzle with honey for a touch of sweetness.

5. Repeat layers as desired.

6. Serve immediately and relish this protein-packed and antioxidant-rich snack.

Nutritional Information (per serving):

- Calories: 200

- Protein: 15g

- Carbohydrates: 20g

- Fiber: 4g

- Fat: 8g

- Potassium: 250mg

- Phosphorus: 150mg

3. Hummus and Veggie Platter

Prep Time: 10 minutes

Cooking Time: 0 minutes

Serving Size: 1 serving

Ingredients:

- 1/2 cup hummus (low-sodium)

- 1 cup mixed veggies (carrot sticks, cucumber slices, bell pepper strips)

- 1 tablespoon olive oil

- 1 teaspoon lemon juice

- Salt and pepper to taste

Instructions:

1. Arrange the mixed veggies on a plate.

2. In a small bowl, mix hummus, olive oil, lemon juice, salt, and pepper to make a dipping sauce.

3. Serve the veggies with the hummus dipping sauce on the side.

4. Enjoy a crunchy, satisfying snack that's rich in fiber and healthy fats.

Nutritional Information (per serving):

- Calories: 180

- Protein: 6g

- Carbohydrates: 15g

- Fiber: 6g

- Fat: 10g

- Potassium: 200mg

- Phosphorus: 120mg

4. Cottage Cheese and Pineapple Bowl

Prep Time: 5 minutes

Cooking Time: 0 minutes

Serving Size: 1 serving

Ingredients:

- 1/2 cup low-fat cottage cheese

- 1/2 cup fresh pineapple chunks

- 1 tablespoon walnuts, chopped

- 1 teaspoon honey (optional)

Instructions:

1. In a bowl, combine cottage cheese and fresh pineapple chunks.

2. Sprinkle chopped walnuts on top for added texture.

3. Optionally, drizzle with honey for sweetness.

4. Mix gently and savor this protein-packed and kidney-friendly snack.

Nutritional Information (per serving):

- Calories: 200

- Protein: 15g

- Carbohydrates: 20g

- Fiber: 2g

- Fat: 8g

- Potassium: 180mg

- Phosphorus: 150mg

5. Baked Sweet Potato Chips

Prep Time: 10 minutes

Cooking Time: 20 minutes

Serving Size: 1 serving

Ingredients:

- 1 medium sweet potato, thinly sliced

- 1 tablespoon olive oil

- 1/2 teaspoon paprika

- 1/2 teaspoon garlic powder

- Salt to taste

Instructions:

1. Preheat the oven to 400°F (200°C).

2. In a bowl, toss sweet potato slices with olive oil, paprika, garlic powder, and salt.

3. Arrange the slices in a single layer on a baking sheet.

4. Bake for 15-20 minutes or until crisp, flipping them halfway through.

5. Allow to cool before serving. Enjoy a crunchy, low-calorie snack.

Nutritional Information (per serving):

- Calories: 120

- Protein: 2g

- Carbohydrates: 20g

- Fiber: 4g

- Fat: 4g

- Potassium: 180mg

- Phosphorus: 50mg

6. Tuna Salad Lettuce Wraps

Prep Time: 15 minutes

Cooking Time: 0 minutes

Serving Size: 2 wraps per serving

Ingredients:

- 1 can tuna in water, drained

- 2 tablespoons mayonnaise (low-fat)

- 1/4 cup celery, finely chopped

- 1 tablespoon red onion, finely chopped

- 1 teaspoon Dijon mustard

- Salt and pepper to taste

- Iceberg lettuce leaves

Instructions:

1. In a bowl, mix tuna, mayonnaise, celery, red onion, Dijon mustard, salt, and pepper.

2. Spoon the tuna mixture onto individual iceberg lettuce leaves.

3. Wrap the leaves to form lettuce wraps.

4. Serve and relish this protein-packed, low-carb snack.

Nutritional Information (per serving):

- Calories: 180

- Protein: 20g

- Carbohydrates: 3g

- Fiber: 1g

- Fat: 10g

- Potassium: 200mg

- Phosphorus: 150mg

7. Roasted Chickpeas

Prep Time: 10 minutes

Cooking Time: 30 minutes

Serving Size: 1/4 cup per serving

Ingredients:

- 1 can chickpeas, drained and rinsed

- 1 tablespoon olive oil

- 1/2 teaspoon cumin

- 1/2 teaspoon paprika

- 1/2 teaspoon garlic powder

- Salt to taste

Instructions:

1. Preheat the oven to 400°F (200°C).

2. Pat chickpeas dry with a paper towel.

3. In a bowl, toss chickpeas with olive oil, cumin, paprika, garlic powder, and salt.

4. Spread the chickpeas in a single layer on a baking sheet.

5. Roast for 25-30 minutes or until golden and crispy.

6. Allow to cool before serving. Enjoy a crunchy, protein-rich snack.

Nutritional Information (per serving):

- Calories: 120

- Protein: 5g

- Carbohydrates: 15g

- Fiber: 4g

- Fat: 4g

- Potassium: 180mg

- Phosphorus: 80mg

8. Veggie and Cheese Skewers

Prep Time: 15 minutes

Cooking Time: 0 minutes

Serving Size: 2 skewers per serving

Ingredients:

- Cherry tomatoes

- Cucumber, cut into chunks

- Bell peppers, cut into squares

- Mozzarella cheese, cubed

- Basil leaves

- Balsamic glaze for drizzling

Instructions:

1. Thread cherry tomatoes, cucumber chunks, bell pepper squares, mozzarella cubes, and basil leaves onto skewers.

2. Arrange the skewers on a serving platter.

3. Drizzle with balsamic glaze before serving.

4. Enjoy this refreshing, low-carb snack with a burst of flavors.

Nutritional Information (per serving):

- Calories: 150

- Protein: 8g

- Carbohydrates: 8g

- Fiber: 2g

- Fat: 10g

- Potassium: 200mg

- Phosphorus: 100mg

9. Egg Salad Lettuce Wraps

Prep Time: 15 minutes

Cooking Time: 10 minutes

Serving Size: 2 wraps per serving

Ingredients:

- 4 hard-boiled eggs, chopped

- 2 tablespoons mayonnaise (low-fat)

- 1 tablespoon Dijon mustard

- 2 tablespoons celery, finely chopped

- Salt and pepper to taste

- Romaine lettuce leaves

Instructions:

1. In a bowl, combine chopped hard-boiled eggs, mayonnaise, Dijon mustard, celery, salt, and pepper.

2. Spoon the egg salad onto individual romaine lettuce leaves.

3. Wrap the leaves to form lettuce wraps.

4. Serve and savor this protein-packed, low-carb snack.

Nutritional Information (per serving):

- Calories: 180

- Protein: 12g

- Carbohydrates: 3g

- Fiber: 1g

- Fat: 14g

- Potassium: 150mg

- Phosphorus: 150mg

10. Berry and Almond Chia Pudding

Prep Time: 5 minutes (plus chilling time)

Cooking Time: 0 minutes

Serving Size: 1 serving

Ingredients:

- 2 tablespoons chia seeds

- 1/2 cup unsweetened almond milk

- 1/4 cup mixed berries (blueberries, raspberries, strawberries)

- 1 tablespoon almonds, sliced

- 1 teaspoon honey (optional)

Instructions:

1. In a jar, combine chia seeds and almond milk. Stir well.

2. Refrigerate for at least 2 hours or overnight to allow the chia seeds to expand.

3. Before serving, top the chia pudding with mixed berries and sliced almonds.

4. Optionally, drizzle with honey for sweetness.

5. Enjoy this delightful, fiber-rich snack that's gentle on both kidneys and blood sugar.

Nutritional Information (per serving):

- Calories: 200

- Protein: 6g

- Carbohydrates: 18g

- Fiber: 10g

- Fat: 12g

- Potassium: 180mg

- Phosphorus: 120mg

SMOOTHIE RECIPES

1. Berry Bliss Smoothie

Prep Time: 5 minutes

Cooking Time: 0 minutes

Serving Size: 1 serving

Ingredients:

- 1/2 cup blueberries (fresh or frozen)

- 1/2 cup strawberries, hulled (fresh or frozen)

- 1/2 banana

- 1/2 cup Greek yogurt (unsweetened)

- 1/2 cup almond milk (unsweetened)

- Ice cubes (optional)

Instructions:

1. Combine blueberries, strawberries, banana, Greek yogurt, and almond milk in a blender.

2. Blend until smooth and creamy.

3. Add ice cubes if a colder consistency is desired.

4. Pour into a glass and enjoy this antioxidant-rich, kidney-friendly smoothie.

Nutritional Information (per serving):

- Calories: 200

- Protein: 15g

- Carbohydrates: 30g

- Fiber: 6g

- Fat: 4g

- Potassium: 300mg

- Phosphorus: 150mg

2. Green Power Smoothie

Prep Time: 7 minutes

Cooking Time: 0 minutes

Serving Size: 1 serving

Ingredients:

- 1 cup spinach leaves

- 1/2 cucumber, peeled and sliced

- 1/2 green apple, cored and diced

- 1/2 lemon, juiced

- 1/2 cup water or coconut water

- Ice cubes (optional)

Instructions:

1. Place spinach leaves, cucumber, green apple, lemon juice, and water in a blender.

2. Blend until smooth, adjusting the consistency with water if needed.

3. Add ice cubes if desired and blend again.

4. Pour into a glass and savor this nutrient-packed, low-sugar smoothie.

Nutritional Information (per serving):

- Calories: 120

- Protein: 4g

- Carbohydrates: 25g

- Fiber: 6g

- Fat: 1g

- Potassium: 300mg

- Phosphorus: 80mg

3. Tropical Paradise Smoothie

Prep Time: 5 minutes

Cooking Time: 0 minutes

Serving Size: 1 serving

Ingredients:

- 1/2 cup pineapple chunks

- 1/2 mango, peeled and diced

- 1/2 banana

- 1/2 cup coconut milk (unsweetened)

- 1/2 cup water

- Ice cubes (optional)

Instructions:

1. Combine pineapple chunks, mango, banana, coconut milk, and water in a blender.

2. Blend until smooth and creamy.

3. Add ice cubes if desired for a refreshing touch.

4. Pour into a glass and enjoy this tropical-inspired, kidney-friendly delight.

Nutritional Information (per serving):

- Calories: 220

- Protein: 2g

- Carbohydrates: 40g

- Fiber: 5g

- Fat: 8g

- Potassium: 300mg

- Phosphorus: 100mg

4. Chocolate Almond Delight Smoothie

Prep Time: 5 minutes

Cooking Time: 0 minutes

Serving Size: 1 serving

Ingredients:

- 1 tablespoon unsweetened cocoa powder

- 1/2 banana

- 1 tablespoon almond butter

- 1/2 cup Greek yogurt (unsweetened)

- 1/2 cup almond milk (unsweetened)

- Ice cubes (optional)

Instructions:

1. In a blender, combine cocoa powder, banana, almond butter, Greek yogurt, and almond milk.

2. Blend until smooth and creamy.

3. Add ice cubes if a colder consistency is preferred.

4. Pour into a glass and relish this chocolatey, protein-packed treat.

Nutritional Information (per serving):

- Calories: 250

- Protein: 15g

- Carbohydrates: 25g

- Fiber: 6g

- Fat: 10g

- Potassium: 350mg

- Phosphorus: 200mg

5. Berry Citrus Burst Smoothie

Prep Time: 6 minutes

Cooking Time: 0 minutes

Serving Size: 1 serving

Ingredients:

- 1/2 cup blueberries (fresh or frozen)

- 1/2 cup raspberries (fresh or frozen)

- 1/2 orange, peeled and segmented

- 1/2 cup Greek yogurt (unsweetened)

- 1/2 cup water or orange juice

- Ice cubes (optional)

Instructions:

1. Place blueberries, raspberries, orange segments, Greek yogurt, and water (or orange juice) in a blender.

2. Blend until smooth and vibrant.

3. Add ice cubes if desired for a refreshing touch.

4. Pour into a glass and indulge in this vitamin C-packed smoothie.

Nutritional Information (per serving):

- Calories: 180

- Protein: 12g

- Carbohydrates: 30g

- Fiber: 8g

- Fat: 3g

- Potassium: 300mg

- Phosphorus: 150mg

6. Avocado Banana Smoothie

Prep Time: 5 minutes

Cooking Time: 0 minutes

Serving Size: 1 serving

Ingredients:

- 1/2 avocado, peeled and pitted

- 1/2 banana

- 1/2 cup spinach leaves

- 1/2 cup almond milk (unsweetened)

- 1/2 cup water

- Ice cubes (optional)

Instructions:

1. In a blender, combine avocado, banana, spinach leaves, almond milk, and water.

2. Blend until smooth and velvety.

3. Add ice cubes if a colder consistency is preferred.

4. Pour into a glass and enjoy this creamy, nutrient-dense smoothie.

Nutritional Information (per serving):

- Calories: 220

- Protein: 5g

- Carbohydrates: 25g

- Fiber: 8g

- Fat: 15g

- Potassium: 400mg

- Phosphorus: 120mg

7. Cinnamon Apple Pie Smoothie

Prep Time: 7 minutes

Cooking Time: 0 minutes

Serving Size: 1 serving

Ingredients:

- 1/2 apple, cored and diced

- 1/2 teaspoon ground cinnamon

- 1/4 teaspoon nutmeg

- 1/2 cup Greek yogurt (unsweetened)

- 1/2 cup almond milk (unsweetened)

- Ice cubes (optional)

Instructions:

1. Combine diced apple, ground cinnamon, nutmeg, Greek yogurt, and almond milk in a blender.

2. Blend until smooth and aromatic.

3. Add ice cubes if a colder consistency is desired.

4. Pour into a glass and savor this cinnamon-spiced, diabetes-friendly treat.

Nutritional Information (per serving):

- Calories: 180

- Protein: 12g

- Carbohydrates: 30g

- Fiber: 6g

- Fat: 3g

- Potassium: 250mg

- Phosphorus: 150mg

8. Pineapple Coconut Dream Smoothie

Prep Time: 5 minutes

Cooking Time: 0 minutes

Serving Size: 1 serving

Ingredients:

- 1/2 cup pineapple chunks

- 1/2 cup coconut milk (unsweetened)

- 1/2 banana

- 1/4 cup unsweetened shredded coconut

- 1/2 cup water

- Ice cubes (optional)

Instructions:

1. Blend pineapple chunks, coconut milk, banana, shredded coconut, and water in a blender.

2. Blend until smooth and tropical.

3. Add ice cubes if desired for a refreshing touch.

4. Pour into a glass and enjoy this exotic, kidney-friendly smoothie.

Nutritional Information (per serving):

- Calories: 220

- Protein: 3g

- Carbohydrates: 25g

- Fiber: 5g

- Fat: 12g

- Potassium: 300mg

- Phosphorus: 100mg

9. Mocha Almond Protein Smoothie

Prep Time: 7 minutes

Cooking Time: 0 minutes

Serving Size: 1 serving

Ingredients:

- 1/2 cup brewed coffee, cooled

- 1/2 banana

- 1 tablespoon unsweetened cocoa powder

- 1 tablespoon almond butter

- 1/2 cup Greek yogurt (unsweetened)

- 1/2 cup almond milk (unsweetened)

- Ice cubes (optional)

Instructions:

1. In a blender, combine brewed coffee, banana, cocoa powder, almond butter, Greek yogurt, and almond milk.

2. Blend until smooth and energizing.

3. Add ice cubes if a colder consistency is preferred.

4. Pour into a glass and relish this mocha-infused, protein-packed smoothie.

Nutritional Information (per serving):

- Calories: 220

- Protein: 15g

- Carbohydrates: 25g

- Fiber: 6g

- Fat: 9g

- Potassium: 350mg

- Phosphorus: 150mg

10. Minty Green Detox Smoothie

Prep Time: 6 minutes

Cooking Time: 0 minutes

Serving Size: 1 serving

Ingredients:

- 1/2 cup cucumber, peeled and sliced

- 1/2 cup pineapple chunks

- 1/2 lime, juiced

- 1/2 avocado, peeled and pitted

- 1/2 cup spinach leaves

- 1/2 cup coconut water

- Ice cubes (optional)

Instructions:

1. Blend cucumber, pineapple chunks, lime juice, avocado, spinach leaves, and coconut water in a blender.

2. Blend until smooth and refreshing.

3. Add ice cubes if desired for a chilled experience.

4. Pour into a glass and enjoy this detoxifying, nutrient-rich smoothie.

Nutritional Information (per serving):

- Calories: 180

- Protein: 5g

- Carbohydrates: 25g

- Fiber: 8g

- Fat: 10g

- Potassium: 350mg

- Phosphorus: 120mg

BREAKFAST RECIPES

1. Veggie Omelette with Spinach and Feta

Prep Time: 10 minutes

Cooking Time: 10 minutes

Serving Size: 1 omelette

Ingredients:

- 2 large eggs

- 1/4 cup fresh spinach, chopped

- 2 tablespoons feta cheese, crumbled

- 1/4 cup bell peppers, diced

- 1/4 cup cherry tomatoes, halved

- Salt and pepper to taste

- Cooking spray

Instructions:

1. In a bowl, beat the eggs and season with salt and pepper.

2. Heat a non-stick pan over medium heat, coat with cooking spray.

3. Add bell peppers and cherry tomatoes, sauté until softened.

4. Pour beaten eggs over veggies, sprinkle spinach and feta on one side.

5. When the edges set, fold the omelette in half.

6. Cook until eggs are fully set, then serve.

Nutritional Information (per serving):

- Calories: 250

- Protein: 18g

- Carbohydrates: 7g

- Fiber: 2g

- Fat: 16g

- Potassium: 350mg

- Phosphorus: 200mg

2. Quinoa Breakfast Bowl with Berries

Prep Time: 15 minutes

Cooking Time: 15 minutes

Serving Size: 1 bowl

Ingredients:

- 1/2 cup cooked quinoa

- 1/4 cup Greek yogurt (unsweetened)

- 1/2 cup mixed berries (blueberries, strawberries)

- 1 tablespoon almonds, sliced

- 1 teaspoon honey (optional)

- 1/4 teaspoon cinnamon

Instructions:

1. In a bowl, layer cooked quinoa.

2. Top with Greek yogurt, mixed berries, and sliced almonds.

3. Drizzle honey and sprinkle cinnamon.

4. Mix gently and enjoy this protein-packed breakfast bowl.

Nutritional Information (per serving):

- Calories: 280

- Protein: 15g

- Carbohydrates: 35g

- Fiber: 6g

- Fat: 10g

- Potassium: 300mg

- Phosphorus: 180mg

3. Sweet Potato and Turkey Sausage Hash

Prep Time: 15 minutes

Cooking Time: 20 minutes

Serving Size: 1 cup

Ingredients:

- 1/2 cup sweet potatoes, diced

- 2 turkey sausage links, sliced

- 1/4 cup onion, chopped

- 1/4 cup bell peppers, diced

- 1 tablespoon olive oil

- Salt and pepper to taste

- 2 eggs (optional, poached or fried)

Instructions:

1. In a skillet, heat olive oil over medium heat.

2. Add sweet potatoes, turkey sausage, onion, and bell peppers.

3. Sauté until sweet potatoes are tender and sausage is cooked.

4. Season with salt and pepper.

5. If desired, top with poached or fried eggs before serving.

Nutritional Information (per serving):

- Calories: 300

- Protein: 18g

- Carbohydrates: 20g

- Fiber: 3g

- Fat: 15g

- Potassium: 400mg

- Phosphorus: 200mg

4. Overnight Chia Pudding with Almond Milk

Prep Time: 5 minutes (plus chilling time)

Cooking Time: 0 minutes

Serving Size: 1 serving

Ingredients:

- 2 tablespoons chia seeds

- 1/2 cup almond milk (unsweetened)

- 1/4 cup mixed berries (raspberries, blueberries)

- 1 tablespoon walnuts, chopped

- 1 teaspoon honey (optional)

Instructions:

1. In a jar, combine chia seeds and almond milk. Stir well.

2. Refrigerate for at least 2 hours or overnight.

3. Before serving, top with mixed berries, chopped walnuts, and honey if desired.

4. Enjoy this fiber-rich, diabetes-friendly breakfast.

Nutritional Information (per serving):

- Calories: 220

- Protein: 5g

- Carbohydrates: 20g

- Fiber: 10g

- Fat: 15g

- Potassium: 200mg

- Phosphorus: 120mg

5. Egg and Veggie Breakfast Burrito

Prep Time: 10 minutes
Cooking Time: 10 minutes
Serving Size: 1 burrito

Ingredients:

- 2 large eggs, scrambled

- 1/4 cup black beans, drained and rinsed

- 1/4 cup bell peppers, diced

- 2 tablespoons onion, chopped

- 1 whole-wheat tortilla

- 1 tablespoon salsa (optional)

- Cooking spray

Instructions:

1. In a skillet, sauté bell peppers and onions until softened.

2. Add scrambled eggs and black beans, cook until eggs are set.

3. Warm the tortilla and place the egg mixture inside.

4. Optionally, top with salsa before rolling into a burrito.

Nutritional Information (per serving):

- Calories: 280

- Protein: 18g

- Carbohydrates: 30g

- Fiber: 7g

- Fat: 10g

- Potassium: 300mg

- Phosphorus: 180mg

6. Almond Flour Pancakes with Berries

Prep Time: 10 minutes

Cooking Time: 10 minutes

Serving Size: 2 pancakes

Ingredients:

- 1/2 cup almond flour

- 2 eggs

- 1/4 cup almond milk (unsweetened)

- 1/2 teaspoon baking powder

- 1/2 teaspoon vanilla extract

- Mixed berries for topping

- Sugar-free syrup (optional)

Instructions:

1. In a bowl, whisk together almond flour, eggs, almond milk, baking powder, and vanilla extract.

2. Heat a skillet over medium heat, coat with cooking spray.

3. Pour batter onto the skillet to form pancakes.

4. Cook until edges set, then flip and cook the other side.

5. Top with mixed berries and sugar-free syrup if desired.

Nutritional Information (per serving):

- Calories: 280

- Protein: 12g

- Carbohydrates: 10g

- Fiber: 4g

- Fat: 22g

- Potassium: 200mg

- Phosphorus: 120mg

7. Avocado Toast with Poached Egg

Prep Time: 10 minutes

Cooking Time: 5 minutes

Serving Size: 1 serving

Ingredients:

- 1 slice whole-grain bread, toasted

- 1/2 avocado, mashed

- 1 large egg, poached

- Salt and pepper to taste

- Red pepper flakes (optional)

Instructions:

1. Toast the whole-grain bread slice.

2. Spread mashed avocado on the toast.

3. Top with a poached egg.

4. Season with salt, pepper, and red pepper flakes if desired.

5. Enjoy this simple, nutritious breakfast.

Nutritional Information (per serving):

- Calories: 250

- Protein: 12g

- Carbohydrates: 20g

- Fiber: 8g

- Fat: 15g

- Potassium: 300mg

- Phosphorus: 180mg

8. Greek Yogurt Parfait with Granola

Prep Time: 5 minutes
Cooking Time: 0 minutes
Serving Size: 1 serving

Ingredients:

- 1/2 cup Greek yogurt (unsweetened)

- 1/4 cup granola (low-sugar)

- 1/4 cup mixed berries (strawberries, blueberries)

- 1 tablespoon honey (optional)

Instructions:

1. In a glass or bowl, layer Greek yogurt at the bottom.

2. Add a layer of granola and then a layer of mixed berries.

3. Optionally, drizzle with honey for sweetness.

4. Repeat layers as desired.

5. Enjoy this protein-packed and antioxidant-rich parfait.

Nutritional Information (per serving):

- Calories: 280

- Protein: 15g

- Carbohydrates: 30g

- Fiber: 4g

- Fat: 12g

- Potassium: 300mg

- Phosphorus: 180mg

9. Smoked Salmon and Cream Cheese Bagel

Prep Time: 10 minutes

Cooking Time: 0 minutes

Serving Size: 1 serving

Ingredients:

- 1 whole-grain bagel, toasted

- 2 tablespoons cream cheese (low-fat)

- 2 ounces smoked salmon

- 1 tablespoon capers

- Fresh dill for garnish

Instructions:

1. Toast the whole-grain bagel.

2. Spread cream cheese on each half.

3. Layer with smoked salmon and sprinkle capers.

4. Garnish with fresh dill.

5. Enjoy this delicious and omega-3 rich breakfast.

Nutritional Information (per serving):

- Calories: 320

- Protein: 18g

- Carbohydrates: 40g

- Fiber: 6g

- Fat: 10g

- Potassium: 350mg

- Phosphorus: 200mg

10. Cinnamon Raisin Oatmeal with Walnuts

Prep Time: 5 minutes

Cooking Time: 5 minutes

Serving Size: 1 serving

Ingredients:

- 1/2 cup rolled oats

- 1/2 cup almond milk (unsweetened)

- 1/4 cup raisins

- 1/2 teaspoon cinnamon

- 1 tablespoon walnuts, chopped

- 1 teaspoon maple syrup (optional)

Instructions:

1. In a saucepan, combine rolled oats, almond milk, raisins, and cinnamon.

2. Cook over medium heat until oats are tender.

3. Top with chopped walnuts and drizzle with maple syrup if desired.

4. Enjoy this warm and comforting oatmeal.

Nutritional Information (per serving):

- Calories: 280

- Protein: 8g

- Carbohydrates: 40g

- Fiber: 6g

- Fat: 10g

- Potassium: 250mg

- Phosphorus: 150mg

11. Spinach and Mushroom Breakfast Wrap

Prep Time: 10 minutes

Cooking Time: 10 minutes

Serving Size: 1 wrap

Ingredients:

- 1 whole-wheat tortilla

- 2 large eggs, scrambled

- 1/2 cup spinach, chopped

- 1/4 cup mushrooms, sliced

- 1/4 cup feta cheese, crumbled

- Salt and pepper to taste

- Cooking spray

Instructions:

1. In a skillet, sauté mushrooms and spinach until wilted.

2. Season with salt and pepper.

3. In a separate pan, scramble eggs until cooked.

4. Warm the tortilla, then assemble with eggs, spinach, mushrooms, and feta.

5. Roll into a wrap and serve.

Nutritional Information (per serving):

- Calories: 320

- Protein: 18g

- Carbohydrates: 25g

- Fiber: 5g

- Fat: 15g

- Potassium: 350mg

- Phosphorus: 200mg

12. Blueberry Almond Butter Smoothie Bowl

Prep Time: 10 minutes

Cooking Time: 0 minutes

Serving Size: 1 bowl

Ingredients:

- 1/2 cup blueberries (fresh or frozen)

- 1/2 banana

- 1/4 cup almond butter

- 1/2 cup almond milk (unsweetened)

- 1/4 cup granola (low-sugar)

- 1 tablespoon chia seeds

Instructions:

1. In a blender, combine blueberries, banana, almond butter, and almond milk.

2. Blend until smooth and creamy.

3. Pour into a bowl and top with granola and chia seeds.

4. Enjoy this nutrient-packed and satisfying smoothie bowl.

Nutritional Information (per serving):

- Calories: 350

- Protein: 12g

- Carbohydrates: 35g

- Fiber: 8g

- Fat: 18g

- Potassium: 300mg

- Phosphorus: 150mg

13. Turkey and Veggie Breakfast Skillet

Prep Time: 15 minutes

Cooking Time: 15 minutes

Serving Size: 1 serving

Ingredients:

- 1/2 cup ground turkey

- 1/4 cup bell peppers, diced

- 1/4 cup onion, chopped

- 1/2 cup sweet potatoes, diced

- 1 tablespoon olive oil

- 2 large eggs

- Salt and pepper to taste

Instructions:

1. In a skillet, heat olive oil over medium heat.

2. Add ground turkey and cook until browned.

3. Add bell peppers, onion, and sweet potatoes. Sauté until veggies are tender.

4. Make two wells in the mixture and crack eggs into them.

5. Cover and cook until eggs are done to your liking.

6. Season with salt and pepper before serving.

Nutritional Information (per serving):

- Calories: 320

- Protein: 20g

- Carbohydrates: 20g

- Fiber: 4g

- Fat: 18g

- Potassium: 400mg

- Phosphorus: 250mg

14. Peanut Butter Banana Breakfast Wrap

Prep Time: 5 minutes

Cooking Time: 5 minutes

Serving Size: 1 wrap

Ingredients:

- 1 whole-wheat tortilla

- 2 tablespoons peanut butter (unsweetened)

- 1 banana, sliced

- 1 tablespoon chia seeds

Instructions:

1. Warm the whole-wheat tortilla.

2. Spread peanut butter over the tortilla.

3. Place banana slices on one half and sprinkle with chia seeds.

4. Fold the tortilla in half, creating a wrap.

5. Slice in half and enjoy this simple yet satisfying breakfast.

Nutritional Information (per serving):

- Calories: 350

- Protein: 10g

- Carbohydrates: 40g

- Fiber: 7g

- Fat: 18g

- Potassium: 300mg

- Phosphorus: 180mg

15. Mediterranean Egg White Scramble

Prep Time: 10 minutes

Cooking Time: 10 minutes

Serving Size: 1 serving

Ingredients:

- 1 cup egg whites

- 1/4 cup cherry tomatoes, halved

- 1/4 cup black olives, sliced

- 2 tablespoons feta cheese, crumbled

- 1 tablespoon fresh basil, chopped

- Salt and pepper to taste

- Cooking spray

Instructions:

1. In a bowl, whisk together egg whites, salt, and pepper.

2. Heat a skillet over medium heat, coat with cooking spray.

3. Pour egg whites into the skillet.

4. Add cherry tomatoes, black olives, and feta cheese.

5. Stir gently until eggs are cooked through.

6. Top with fresh basil before serving.

Nutritional Information (per serving):

- Calories: 220

- Protein: 30g

- Carbohydrates: 8g

- Fiber: 2g

- Fat: 8g

- Potassium: 300mg

- Phosphorus: 200mg

16. Banana Walnut Breakfast Muffins

Prep Time: 15 minutes

Cooking Time: 20 minutes

Serving Size: 2 muffins

Ingredients:

- 1 cup whole wheat flour

- 1/2 cup rolled oats

- 1 teaspoon baking powder

- 1/2 teaspoon baking soda

- 1/4 cup coconut oil, melted

- 1/4 cup honey

- 2 large bananas, mashed

- 1/4 cup walnuts, chopped

- 2 eggs

- 1/2 cup almond milk (unsweetened)

Instructions:

1. Preheat the oven to 350°F (180°C). Line a muffin tin with paper liners.

2. In a bowl, mix whole wheat flour, rolled oats, baking powder, and baking soda.

3. In a separate bowl, whisk together melted coconut oil, honey, mashed bananas, eggs, and almond milk.

4. Combine wet and dry ingredients, fold in chopped walnuts.

5. Divide the batter into muffin cups and bake for 20 minutes or until a toothpick comes out clean.

Nutritional Information (per serving - 2 muffins):

- Calories: 280

- Protein: 8g

- Carbohydrates: 40g

- Fiber: 6g

- Fat: 12g

- Potassium: 250mg

- Phosphorus: 150mg

17. Tomato and Basil Avocado Toast

Prep Time: 10 minutes

Cooking Time: 5 minutes

Serving Size: 1 serving

Ingredients:

- 1 slice whole-grain bread, toasted

- 1/2 avocado, mashed

- 1/2 cup cherry tomatoes, halved

- Fresh basil leaves

- Balsamic glaze for drizzling

Instructions:

1. Toast the whole-grain bread slice.

2. Spread mashed avocado on the toast.

3. Arrange halved cherry tomatoes on top.

4. Garnish with fresh basil leaves.

5. Drizzle with balsamic glaze before serving.

Nutritional Information (per serving):

- Calories: 270

- Protein: 8g

- Carbohydrates: 30g

- Fiber: 8g

- Fat: 15g

- Potassium: 400mg

- Phosphorus: 150mg

18. Chickpea and Spinach Breakfast Bowl

Prep Time: 10 minutes
Cooking Time: 10 minutes
Serving Size: 1 bowl

Ingredients:

- 1/2 cup canned chickpeas, drained and rinsed

- 1 cup fresh spinach

- 1/4 cup red bell pepper, diced

- 1 tablespoon olive oil

- 1 clove garlic, minced

- 1/2 teaspoon cumin

- Salt and pepper to taste

- 1 poached egg

Instructions:

1. In a skillet, heat olive oil over medium heat.

2. Add minced garlic and sauté until fragrant.

3. Add chickpeas, cumin, salt, and pepper. Cook until chickpeas are golden.

4. Add fresh spinach and red bell pepper, cook until spinach wilts.

5. Top with a poached egg before serving.

Nutritional Information (per serving):

- Calories: 320

- Protein: 16g

- Carbohydrates: 30g

- Fiber: 8g

- Fat: 15g

- Potassium: 350mg

- Phosphorus: 200mg

19. Pecan and Apple Cinnamon Pancakes

Prep Time: 15 minutes

Cooking Time: 10 minutes

Serving Size: 2 pancakes

Ingredients:

- 1/2 cup oat flour

- 1/2 teaspoon baking powder

- 1/2 teaspoon cinnamon

- 1/2 cup almond milk (unsweetened)

- 1/2 apple, grated

- 2 tablespoons chopped pecans

- 1 tablespoon maple syrup

Instructions:

1. In a bowl, mix oat flour, baking powder, and cinnamon.

2. Add almond milk, grated apple, and chopped pecans. Stir until combined.

3. Heat a skillet over medium heat, coat with cooking spray.

4. Pour batter onto the skillet to form pancakes.

5. Cook until edges set, then flip and cook the other side.

6. Drizzle with maple syrup before serving.

Nutritional Information (per serving):

- Calories: 300

- Protein: 8g

- Carbohydrates: 40g

- Fiber: 6g

- Fat: 12g

- Potassium: 250mg

- Phosphorus: 150mg

20. Berry and Spinach Breakfast Smoothie

Prep Time: 5 minutes

Cooking Time: 0 minutes

Serving Size: 1 smoothie

Ingredients:

- 1/2 cup mixed berries (strawberries, blueberries, raspberries)

- 1/2 banana

- Handful of fresh spinach

- 1/2 cup Greek yogurt (unsweetened)

- 1/2 cup almond milk (unsweetened)

- 1 tablespoon chia seeds

Instructions:

1. In a blender, combine mixed berries, banana, spinach, Greek yogurt, and almond milk.

2. Blend until smooth and creamy.

3. Pour into a glass and top with chia seeds.

4. Enjoy this antioxidant-rich and nutrient-packed breakfast smoothie.

Nutritional Information (per serving):

- Calories: 280

- Protein: 15g

- Carbohydrates: 35g

- Fiber: 8g

- Fat: 12g

- Potassium: 300mg

- Phosphorus: 150mg

LUNCH RECIPES

1. Grilled Chicken Salad with Balsamic Vinaigrette

Prep Time: 15 minutes

Cooking Time: 15 minutes

Serving Size: 1 salad

Ingredients:

- 4 oz grilled chicken breast, sliced

- 2 cups mixed salad greens

- 1/2 cup cherry tomatoes, halved

- 1/4 cup cucumber, sliced

- 1/4 cup red bell pepper, diced

- 2 tablespoons feta cheese, crumbled

- 1 tablespoon balsamic vinaigrette dressing

Instructions:

1. Grill chicken breast until fully cooked, then slice.

2. In a bowl, combine salad greens, cherry tomatoes, cucumber, red bell pepper, and grilled chicken.

3. Sprinkle feta cheese on top.

4. Drizzle with balsamic vinaigrette dressing and toss gently.

5. Enjoy this nutritious and protein-packed chicken salad.

Nutritional Information (per serving):

- Calories: 300

- Protein: 30g

- Carbohydrates: 15g

- Fiber: 5g

- Fat: 12g

- Potassium: 400mg

- Phosphorus: 250mg

2. Quinoa and Black Bean Bowl

Prep Time: 20 minutes

Cooking Time: 15 minutes

Serving Size: 1 bowl

Ingredients:

- 1/2 cup cooked quinoa

- 1/2 cup black beans, cooked and drained

- 1/4 cup corn kernels (fresh or frozen)

- 1/4 cup red onion, finely chopped

- 1/4 cup avocado, diced

- 1 tablespoon cilantro, chopped

- 1 tablespoon lime juice

- Salt and pepper to taste

Instructions:

1. Cook quinoa according to package instructions.

2. In a bowl, combine cooked quinoa, black beans, corn, red onion, avocado, and cilantro.

3. Drizzle with lime juice and season with salt and pepper.

4. Mix well and savor this protein and fiber-rich bowl.

Nutritional Information (per serving):

- Calories: 280

- Protein: 15g

- Carbohydrates: 40g

- Fiber: 8g

- Fat: 10g

- Potassium: 350mg

- Phosphorus: 200mg

3. Salmon and Asparagus Foil Packets

Prep Time: 10 minutes

Cooking Time: 20 minutes

Serving Size: 1 packet

Ingredients:

- 6 oz salmon fillet

- 1/2 cup asparagus, trimmed

- 1/4 cup cherry tomatoes, halved

- 1 tablespoon olive oil

- 1 clove garlic, minced

- Lemon slices

- Fresh dill for garnish

- Salt and pepper to taste

Instructions:

1. Preheat the oven to 400°F (200°C).

2. Place a piece of foil on a baking sheet.

3. In the center, lay salmon fillet, asparagus, and cherry tomatoes.

4. Drizzle with olive oil, sprinkle minced garlic, salt, and pepper.

5. Seal the foil packet tightly and bake for 20 minutes.

6. Garnish with lemon slices and fresh dill before serving.

Nutritional Information (per serving):

- Calories: 350

- Protein: 25g

- Carbohydrates: 8g

- Fiber: 3g

- Fat: 20g

- Potassium: 450mg

- Phosphorus: 250mg

4. Lentil and Vegetable Stir-Fry

Prep Time: 15 minutes
Cooking Time: 20 minutes
Serving Size: 1 stir-fry

Ingredients:

- 1/2 cup dry lentils, cooked

- 1 cup broccoli florets

- 1/2 cup bell peppers, sliced

- 1/4 cup carrots, julienned

- 2 tablespoons soy sauce (low-sodium)

- 1 tablespoon sesame oil

- 1 clove garlic, minced

- 1 teaspoon ginger, grated

- Green onions for garnish

- Brown rice (optional, for serving)

Instructions:

1. Cook lentils according to package instructions.

2. In a wok or skillet, heat sesame oil over medium-high heat.

3. Add garlic and ginger, sauté for a minute.

4. Stir in broccoli, bell peppers, and carrots. Cook until vegetables are tender-crisp.

5. Add cooked lentils and soy sauce, toss to combine.

6. Garnish with green onions and serve over brown rice if desired.

Nutritional Information (per serving):

- Calories: 320

- Protein: 18g

- Carbohydrates: 40g

- Fiber: 12g

- Fat: 10g

- Potassium: 500mg

- Phosphorus: 300mg

5. Turkey and Vegetable Skewers

Prep Time: 15 minutes

Cooking Time: 15 minutes

Serving Size: 2 skewers

Ingredients:

- 6 oz turkey breast, cut into cubes

- 1/2 cup cherry tomatoes

- 1/2 cup bell peppers, diced

- 1/4 cup red onion, cut into chunks

- 1 tablespoon olive oil

- 1 teaspoon dried oregano

- 1 teaspoon smoked paprika

- Salt and pepper to taste

- Wooden skewers, soaked in water

Instructions:

1. Preheat the grill or grill pan over medium-high heat.

2. In a bowl, combine turkey cubes, cherry tomatoes, bell peppers, red onion, olive oil, oregano, smoked paprika, salt, and pepper.

3. Thread the marinated ingredients onto soaked wooden skewers.

4. Grill for 12-15 minutes, turning occasionally, until turkey is cooked through.

5. Serve these flavorful skewers on a bed of quinoa or with a side salad.

Nutritional Information (per serving):

- Calories: 280

- Protein: 30g

- Carbohydrates: 15g

- Fiber: 4g

- Fat: 12g

- Potassium: 400mg

- Phosphorus: 250mg

6. Eggplant and Chickpea Curry

Prep Time: 20 minutes

Cooking Time: 25 minutes

Serving Size: 1 curry bowl

Ingredients:

- 1 cup eggplant, diced

- 1/2 cup canned chickpeas, drained and rinsed

- 1/2 cup tomatoes, diced

- 1/4 cup onion, finely chopped

- 2 cloves garlic, minced

- 1 teaspoon curry powder

- 1/2 teaspoon turmeric

- 1/2 teaspoon cumin

- 1/4 teaspoon cayenne pepper (optional)

- 1 tablespoon olive oil

- 1/2 cup vegetable broth

- Fresh cilantro for garnish

- Brown rice (optional, for serving)

Instructions:

1. In a skillet, heat olive oil over medium heat.

2. Add onion and garlic, sauté until softened.

3. Stir in eggplant, chickpeas, tomatoes, curry powder, turmeric, cumin, and cayenne pepper.

4. Pour in vegetable broth, cover, and simmer for 20-25 minutes.

5. Garnish with fresh cilantro and serve over brown rice if desired.

Nutritional Information (per serving):

- Calories: 300

- Protein: 10g

- Carbohydrates: 40g

- Fiber: 12g

- Fat: 12g

- Potassium: 450mg

- Phosphorus: 200mg

7. Shrimp and Zucchini Noodles

Prep Time: 15 minutes

Cooking Time: 10 minutes

Serving Size: 1 serving

Ingredients:

- 6 oz shrimp, peeled and deveined

- 1 medium zucchini, spiralized

- 1/4 cup cherry tomatoes, halved

- 1/4 cup bell peppers, julienned

- 2 tablespoons pesto sauce

- 1 tablespoon olive oil

- Lemon zest for garnish

- Salt and pepper to taste

Instructions:

1. In a skillet, heat olive oil over medium-high heat.

2. Add shrimp and cook until pink and opaque.

3. Stir in zucchini noodles, cherry tomatoes, and bell peppers.

4. Add pesto sauce, toss until well coated and heated through.

5. Season with salt and pepper, garnish with lemon zest before serving.

Nutritional Information (per serving):

- Calories: 320

- Protein: 20g

- Carbohydrates: 10g

- Fiber: 3g

- Fat: 18g

- Potassium: 400mg

- Phosphorus: 250mg

8. Vegetable and Tofu Stir-Fry

Prep Time: 20 minutes
Cooking Time: 15 minutes
Serving Size: 1 stir-fry

Ingredients:

- 1/2 cup extra-firm tofu, cubed

- 1 cup broccoli florets

- 1/2 cup snap peas

- 1/4 cup carrots, sliced

- 2 tablespoons soy sauce (low-sodium)

- 1 tablespoon sesame oil

- 1 clove garlic, minced

- 1 teaspoon ginger, grated

- Brown rice (optional, for serving)

Instructions:

1. Press tofu to remove excess water, then cube.

2. In a wok or skillet, heat sesame oil over medium-high heat.

3. Add garlic and ginger, sauté for a minute.

4. Stir in tofu, broccoli, snap peas, and carrots. Cook until vegetables are tender-crisp.

5. Add soy sauce, toss to combine.

6. Serve over brown rice if desired.

Nutritional Information (per serving):

- Calories: 280

- Protein: 20g

- Carbohydrates: 25g

- Fiber: 8g

- Fat: 15g

- Potassium: 350mg

- Phosphorus: 200mg

9. Spinach and Feta Stuffed Chicken Breast

Prep Time: 15 minutes

Cooking Time: 25 minutes

Serving Size: 1 stuffed chicken breast

Ingredients:

- 6 oz chicken breast

- 1 cup fresh spinach

- 2 tablespoons feta cheese, crumbled

- 1 clove garlic, minced

- 1 teaspoon olive oil

- Lemon wedges for serving

- Salt and pepper to taste

Instructions:

1. Preheat the oven to 375°F (190°C).

2. In a skillet, sauté spinach and garlic in olive oil until wilted.

3. Butterfly the chicken breast and stuff with sautéed spinach and feta.

4. Season with salt and pepper, then secure with toothpicks.

5. Bake for 25 minutes or until chicken is cooked through.

6. Serve with lemon wedges for a burst of freshness.

Nutritional Information (per serving):

- Calories: 280

- Protein: 30g

- Carbohydrates: 5g

- Fiber: 2g

- Fat: 15g

- Potassium: 400mg

- Phosphorus: 250mg

10. Pesto Zoodles with Cherry Tomatoes and Chicken

Prep Time: 20 minutes

Cooking Time: 15 minutes

Serving Size: 1 serving

Ingredients:

- 6 oz chicken breast, cooked and shredded

- 1 medium zucchini, spiralized

- 1/2 cup cherry tomatoes, halved

- 2 tablespoons pesto sauce

- 1 tablespoon olive oil

- Parmesan cheese for garnish

- Salt and pepper to taste

Instructions:

1. In a skillet, heat olive oil over medium-high heat.

2. Add spiralized zucchini and cherry tomatoes, cook until slightly tender.

3. Stir in cooked and shredded chicken.

4. Add pesto sauce, toss until well coated and heated through.

5. Season with salt and pepper, garnish with Parmesan cheese.

Nutritional Information (per serving):

- Calories: 320

- Protein: 25g

- Carbohydrates: 10g

- Fiber: 3g

- Fat: 18g

- Potassium: 400mg

- Phosphorus: 250mg

11. Blackened Tilapia Tacos with Cabbage Slaw

Prep Time: 15 minutes

Cooking Time: 10 minutes

Serving Size: 2 tacos

Ingredients:

- 2 tilapia fillets

- 1 tablespoon blackened seasoning

- 1 cup purple cabbage, shredded

- 1/4 cup plain Greek yogurt (unsweetened)

- 1 tablespoon lime juice

- 1/4 cup cilantro, chopped

- 4 small corn tortillas

- Salsa for topping

Instructions:

1. Rub tilapia fillets with blackened seasoning.

2. Cook tilapia on a grill or skillet for 4-5 minutes per side.

3. In a bowl, mix shredded cabbage, Greek yogurt, lime juice, and cilantro to make the slaw.

4. Warm corn tortillas and assemble tacos with tilapia and cabbage slaw.

5. Top with salsa and enjoy these flavorful tilapia tacos.

Nutritional Information (per serving):

- Calories: 300

- Protein: 25g

- Carbohydrates: 25g

- Fiber: 5g

- Fat: 12g

- Potassium: 450mg

- Phosphorus: 300mg

12. Mediterranean Chickpea Salad

Prep Time: 15 minutes
Cooking Time: 0 minutes
Serving Size: 1 salad

Ingredients:

- 1/2 cup canned chickpeas, drained and rinsed

- 1/2 cup cucumber, diced

- 1/4 cup cherry tomatoes, halved

- 1/4 cup red onion, finely chopped

- 2 tablespoons Kalamata olives, sliced

- 2 tablespoons feta cheese, crumbled

- 1 tablespoon olive oil

- 1 tablespoon balsamic vinegar

- Fresh oregano for garnish

Instructions:

1. In a bowl, combine chickpeas, cucumber, cherry tomatoes, red onion, olives, and feta cheese.

2. Drizzle with olive oil and balsamic vinegar.

3. Toss gently and garnish with fresh oregano.

4. Enjoy this refreshing and satisfying Mediterranean chickpea salad.

Nutritional Information (per serving):

- Calories: 280

- Protein: 10g

- Carbohydrates: 30g

- Fiber: 8g

- Fat: 15g

- Potassium: 350mg

- Phosphorus: 200mg

13. Turkey and Quinoa Stuffed Peppers

Prep Time: 20 minutes

Cooking Time: 25 minutes

Serving Size: 2 stuffed peppers

Ingredients:

- 1/2 cup cooked quinoa

- 1/2 lb ground turkey

- 2 bell peppers, halved and seeds removed

- 1/4 cup black beans, drained and rinsed

- 1/4 cup corn kernels (fresh or frozen)

- 1/4 cup salsa

- 1/4 cup shredded cheddar cheese

- 1 teaspoon taco seasoning

- Fresh cilantro for garnish

Instructions:

1. Preheat the oven to 375°F (190°C).

2. In a skillet, cook ground turkey until browned.

3. Stir in cooked quinoa, black beans, corn, salsa, and taco seasoning.

4. Fill halved bell peppers with the turkey and quinoa mixture.

5. Top with shredded cheddar cheese and bake for 20-25 minutes.

6. Garnish with fresh cilantro before serving.

Nutritional Information (per serving):

- Calories: 320

- Protein: 25g

- Carbohydrates: 25g

- Fiber: 5g

- Fat: 15g

- Potassium: 400mg

- Phosphorus: 250mg

14. Broccoli and Cheddar Stuffed Baked Potatoes

Prep Time: 15 minutes

Cooking Time: 1 hour

Serving Size: 1 stuffed baked potato

Ingredients:

- 1 large baked potato

- 1 cup broccoli florets, steamed

- 1/4 cup cheddar cheese, shredded

- 2 tablespoons Greek yogurt (unsweetened)

- 1 tablespoon chives, chopped

- Salt and pepper to taste

Instructions:

1. Bake the potato until tender (about 45-60 minutes).

2. Cut the top of the potato and scoop out some of the flesh.

3. Mash the removed potato flesh with Greek yogurt, salt, and pepper.

4. Steam broccoli florets and mix with the mashed potato.

5. Spoon the mixture back into the potato skin.

6. Top with shredded cheddar cheese and chives.

7. Broil for a few minutes until cheese is melted and bubbly.

Nutritional Information (per serving):

- Calories: 280

- Protein: 10g

- Carbohydrates: 40g

- Fiber: 6g

- Fat: 10g

- Potassium: 450mg

- Phosphorus: 250mg

15. Caprese Chicken Skillet

Prep Time: 15 minutes

Cooking Time: 20 minutes

Serving Size: 1 chicken breast

Ingredients:

- 1 boneless, skinless chicken breast

- 1/2 cup cherry tomatoes, halved

- 1/4 cup fresh mozzarella, sliced

- 2 tablespoons balsamic glaze

- Fresh basil leaves for garnish

- Salt and pepper to taste

Instructions:

1. Season chicken breast with salt and pepper.

2. In a skillet, cook chicken over medium heat until no longer pink.

3. Top with cherry tomatoes and mozzarella slices.

4. Cover the skillet until cheese is melted and tomatoes are warmed.

5. Drizzle with balsamic glaze and garnish with fresh basil.

Nutritional Information (per serving):

- Calories: 300

- Protein: 30g

- Carbohydrates: 8g

- Fiber: 2g

- Fat: 15g

- Potassium: 400mg

- Phosphorus: 250mg

16. Cauliflower Fried Rice with Shrimp

Prep Time: 20 minutes

Cooking Time: 15 minutes

Serving Size: 1 serving

Ingredients:

- 6 oz shrimp, peeled and deveined

- 1 cup cauliflower rice

- 1/4 cup carrots, diced

- 1/4 cup peas

- 1/4 cup scallions, chopped

- 1 clove garlic, minced

- 1 tablespoon soy sauce (low-sodium)

- 1 tablespoon sesame oil

- 1 egg, beaten

- Sesame seeds for garnish

Instructions:

1. In a wok or skillet, heat sesame oil over medium-high heat.

2. Add shrimp and cook until pink and opaque.

3. Push shrimp to the side and add minced garlic.

4. Stir in cauliflower rice, carrots, peas, and scallions. Cook until vegetables are tender.

5. Push the mixture to the side and pour the beaten egg into the empty space.

6. Scramble the egg until cooked and mix it into the rice mixture.

7. Add soy sauce, toss well, and garnish with sesame seeds.

Nutritional Information (per serving):

- Calories: 320

- Protein: 25g

- Carbohydrates: 20g

- Fiber: 6g

- Fat: 15g

- Potassium: 400mg

- Phosphorus: 250mg

17. Chicken and Vegetable Kebabs

Prep Time: 20 minutes

Cooking Time: 15 minutes

Serving Size: 2 kebabs

Ingredients:

- 6 oz chicken breast, cut into cubes

- 1/2 cup cherry tomatoes

- 1/2 cup zucchini, sliced

- 1/4 cup red onion, cut into chunks

- 1/4 cup bell peppers, diced

- 1 tablespoon olive oil

- 1 teaspoon Italian seasoning

- Salt and pepper to taste

- Wooden skewers, soaked in water

Instructions:

1. Preheat the grill or grill pan over medium-high heat.

2. In a bowl, combine chicken cubes, cherry tomatoes, zucchini, red onion, bell peppers, olive oil, Italian seasoning, salt, and pepper.

3. Thread the marinated ingredients onto soaked wooden skewers.

4. Grill for 12-15 minutes, turning occasionally, until chicken is cooked through.

5. Serve these flavorful kebabs with a side of quinoa or a green salad.

Nutritional Information (per serving):

- Calories: 280

- Protein: 30g

- Carbohydrates: 15g

- Fiber: 4g

- Fat: 12g

- Potassium: 400mg

- Phosphorus: 250mg

18. Ratatouille with Chicken

Prep Time: 20 minutes

Cooking Time: 25 minutes

Serving Size: 1 serving

Ingredients:

- 6 oz chicken thigh, boneless and skinless

- 1/2 cup eggplant, diced

- 1/2 cup zucchini, diced

- 1/2 cup bell peppers, diced

- 1/2 cup tomatoes, diced

- 1/4 cup onion, finely chopped

- 2 cloves garlic, minced

- 1 tablespoon olive oil

- 1 teaspoon dried thyme

- Salt and pepper to taste

Instructions:

1. Season chicken thigh with salt and pepper.

2. In a skillet, heat olive oil over medium-high heat.

3. Cook chicken until browned on both sides and cooked through.

4. Remove chicken and set aside.

5. In the same skillet, sauté garlic and onion until softened.

6. Add eggplant, zucchini, bell peppers, and tomatoes. Cook until vegetables are tender.

7. Stir in dried thyme and return cooked chicken to the skillet.

8. Simmer for a few minutes until flavors meld together.

Nutritional Information (per serving):

- Calories: 320

- Protein: 25g

- Carbohydrates: 20g

- Fiber: 6g

- Fat: 15g

- Potassium: 450mg

- Phosphorus: 250mg

19. Turkey and Sweet Potato Hash

Prep Time: 20 minutes

Cooking Time: 20 minutes

Serving Size: 1 serving

Ingredients:

- 1/2 lb ground turkey

- 1 medium sweet potato, diced

- 1/4 cup red bell pepper, diced

- 1/4 cup red onion, finely chopped

- 1 clove garlic, minced

- 1 tablespoon olive oil

- 1 teaspoon paprika

- 1/2 teaspoon cumin

- Salt and pepper to taste

- Fresh parsley for garnish

Instructions:

1. In a skillet, heat olive oil over medium heat.

2. Add ground turkey and cook until browned.

3. Stir in sweet potato, red bell pepper, red onion, and garlic.

4. Season with paprika, cumin, salt, and pepper.

5. Cook until sweet potatoes are tender.

6. Garnish with fresh parsley before serving.

Nutritional Information (per serving):

- Calories: 300

- Protein: 20g

- Carbohydrates: 30g

- Fiber: 6g

- Fat: 15g

- Potassium: 400mg

- Phosphorus: 250mg

20. Spinach and Mushroom Stuffed Chicken Breast

Prep Time: 20 minutes

Cooking Time: 25 minutes

Serving Size: 1 stuffed chicken breast

Ingredients:

- 6 oz chicken breast

- 1/2 cup spinach, chopped

- 1/4 cup mushrooms, sliced

- 2 tablespoons feta cheese, crumbled

- 1 clove garlic, minced

- 1 teaspoon olive oil

- Lemon wedges for serving

- Salt and pepper to taste

Instructions:

1. Preheat the oven to 375°F (190°C).

2. In a skillet, sauté mushrooms, garlic, and spinach in olive oil until wilted.

3. Butterfly the chicken breast and stuff with sautéed spinach, mushrooms, and feta.

4. Season with salt and pepper, then secure with toothpicks.

5. Bake for 25 minutes or until chicken is cooked through.

6. Serve with lemon wedges for a burst of freshness.

Nutritional Information (per serving):

- Calories: 280

- Protein: 30g

- Carbohydrates: 5g

- Fiber: 2g

- Fat: 15g

- Potassium: 400mg

- Phosphorus: 250mg

DINNER RECIPES

1. Baked Salmon with Lemon-Dill Sauce

Prep Time: 15 minutes

Cooking Time: 20 minutes

Serving Size: 1 fillet

Ingredients:

- 6 oz salmon fillet

- 1 tablespoon olive oil

- 1 tablespoon fresh dill, chopped

- 1 clove garlic, minced

- 1 tablespoon lemon juice

- Salt and pepper to taste

Instructions:

1. Preheat the oven to 375°F (190°C).

2. Place the salmon fillet on a baking sheet.

3. In a bowl, mix olive oil, dill, garlic, lemon juice, salt, and pepper.

4. Brush the salmon with the mixture.

5. Bake for 20 minutes or until the salmon flakes easily with a fork.

6. Serve with additional lemon slices.

Nutritional Information (per serving):

- Calories: 350

- Protein: 30g

- Carbohydrates: 0g

- Fiber: 0g

- Fat: 25g

- Potassium: 450mg

- Phosphorus: 300mg

2. Quinoa-Stuffed Bell Peppers

Prep Time: 20 minutes
Cooking Time: 25 minutes
Serving Size: 2 stuffed peppers

Ingredients:

- 1 cup cooked quinoa

- 1/2 lb ground turkey

- 2 bell peppers, halved and seeds removed

- 1/4 cup black beans, drained and rinsed

- 1/4 cup corn kernels (fresh or frozen)

- 1/4 cup salsa

- 1/4 cup shredded cheddar cheese

- 1 teaspoon taco seasoning

- Fresh cilantro for garnish

Instructions:

1. Preheat the oven to 375°F (190°C).

2. In a skillet, cook ground turkey until browned.

3. Stir in cooked quinoa, black beans, corn, salsa, and taco seasoning.

4. Fill halved bell peppers with the turkey and quinoa mixture.

5. Top with shredded cheddar cheese and bake for 20-25 minutes.

6. Garnish with fresh cilantro before serving.

Nutritional Information (per serving):

- Calories: 320

- Protein: 25g

- Carbohydrates: 25g

- Fiber: 5g

- Fat: 15g

- Potassium: 400mg

- Phosphorus: 250mg

3. Chicken and Vegetable Stir-Fry with Brown Rice

Prep Time: 20 minutes
Cooking Time: 15 minutes
Serving Size: 1 stir-fry

Ingredients:

- 6 oz chicken breast, sliced

- 1/2 cup broccoli florets

- 1/2 cup snap peas

- 1/4 cup carrots, sliced

- 2 tablespoons soy sauce (low-sodium)

- 1 tablespoon sesame oil

- 1 clove garlic, minced

- 1 teaspoon ginger, grated

- Brown rice (cooked, for serving)

Instructions:

1. In a wok or skillet, heat sesame oil over medium-high heat.

2. Add garlic and ginger, sauté for a minute.

3. Stir in chicken, broccoli, snap peas, and carrots. Cook until chicken is browned.

4. Add soy sauce, toss to combine.

5. Serve over cooked brown rice.

Nutritional Information (per serving):

- Calories: 350

- Protein: 30g

- Carbohydrates: 30g

- Fiber: 6g

- Fat: 15g

- Potassium: 500mg

- Phosphorus: 300mg

4. Lentil Soup with Spinach and Tomatoes

Prep Time: 15 minutes

Cooking Time: 30 minutes

Serving Size: 1 bowl

Ingredients:

- 1/2 cup dry lentils, rinsed
- 1 cup spinach, chopped
- 1/2 cup tomatoes, diced
- 1/4 cup onion, finely chopped
- 1 carrot, diced
- 1 celery stalk, diced
- 2 cloves garlic, minced
- 4 cups low-sodium vegetable broth
- 1 teaspoon cumin
- 1/2 teaspoon coriander
- Salt and pepper to taste

Instructions:

1. In a pot, sauté onion and garlic until softened.
2. Add lentils, tomatoes, carrot, celery, cumin, coriander, salt, and pepper.
3. Pour in vegetable broth and bring to a boil.
4. Reduce heat and simmer for 25-30 minutes until lentils are tender.
5. Stir in chopped spinach just before serving.

Nutritional Information (per serving):

- Calories: 300

- Protein: 20g

- Carbohydrates: 50g

- Fiber: 15g

- Fat: 5g

- Potassium: 600mg

- Phosphorus: 250mg

5. Eggplant and Chickpea Curry

Prep Time: 20 minutes
Cooking Time: 25 minutes
Serving Size: 1 serving

Ingredients:

- 1 cup eggplant, diced

- 1/2 cup chickpeas, cooked

- 1/2 cup tomatoes, diced

- 1/4 cup onion, finely chopped

- 2 cloves garlic, minced

- 1 tablespoon curry powder

- 1 teaspoon cumin

- 1/2 teaspoon turmeric

- 1/4 teaspoon cayenne pepper

- 1 cup coconut milk (unsweetened)

- Fresh cilantro for garnish

- Brown rice (cooked, for serving)

Instructions:

1. In a skillet, sauté onion and garlic until translucent.

2. Add eggplant, chickpeas, tomatoes, curry powder, cumin, turmeric, and cayenne pepper.

3. Pour in coconut milk and simmer for 20-25 minutes.

4. Garnish with fresh cilantro and serve over cooked brown rice.

Nutritional Information (per serving):

- Calories: 350

- Protein: 15g

- Carbohydrates: 40g

- Fiber: 10g

- Fat: 18g

- Potassium: 500mg

- Phosphorus: 200mg

6. Turkey and Vegetable Skewers with Quinoa

Prep Time: 20 minutes

Cooking Time: 15 minutes

Serving Size: 2 skewers

Ingredients:

- 1/2 lb ground turkey

- 1/2 cup zucchini, sliced

- 1/2 cup cherry tomatoes

- 1/4 cup red onion, cut into chunks

- 1/4 cup bell peppers, diced

- 1 cup cooked quinoa

- 1 tablespoon olive oil

- 1 teaspoon Italian seasoning

- Salt and pepper to taste

Instructions:

1. Preheat the grill or grill pan over medium-high heat.

2. In a bowl, mix ground turkey with Italian seasoning, salt, and pepper.

3. Thread turkey, zucchini, cherry tomatoes, red onion, and bell peppers onto skewers.

4. Grill for 12-15 minutes, turning occasionally, until turkey is cooked through.

5. Serve over a bed of cooked quinoa.

Nutritional Information (per serving):

- Calories: 320

- Protein: 25g

- Carbohydrates: 30g

- Fiber: 5g

- Fat: 15g

- Potassium: 450mg

- Phosphorus: 250mg

7. Chickpea and Spinach Stew

Prep Time: 15 minutes

Cooking Time: 25 minutes

Serving Size: 1 bowl

Ingredients:

- 1/2 cup canned chickpeas, drained and rinsed

- 2 cups spinach, chopped

- 1/2 cup tomatoes, diced

- 1/4 cup onion, finely chopped

- 2 cloves garlic, minced

- 1 cup low-sodium vegetable broth

- 1 teaspoon smoked paprika

- 1/2 teaspoon cumin

- Salt and pepper to taste

- Lemon wedges for serving

Instructions:

1. In a pot, sauté onion and garlic until softened.

2. Add chickpeas, tomatoes, smoked paprika, cumin, salt, and pepper.

3. Pour in vegetable broth and bring to a simmer.

4. Add chopped spinach and cook until wilted.

5. Serve with a squeeze of fresh lemon.

Nutritional Information (per serving):

- Calories: 280

- Protein: 15g

- Carbohydrates: 45g

- Fiber: 12g

- Fat: 5g

- Potassium: 550mg

- Phosphorus: 200mg

8. Stuffed Acorn Squash with Ground Beef

Prep Time: 20 minutes

Cooking Time: 40 minutes

Serving Size: 1/2 stuffed squash

Ingredients:

- 1 acorn squash, halved and seeds removed

- 1/2 lb lean ground beef

- 1/2 cup quinoa, cooked

- 1/4 cup cranberries, dried

- 1/4 cup pecans, chopped

- 1/4 cup feta cheese, crumbled

- 1 teaspoon cinnamon

- Salt and pepper to taste

Instructions:

1. Preheat the oven to 375°F (190°C).

2. Place acorn squash halves on a baking sheet, cut side down.

3. Bake for 20 minutes, then flip the squash over.

4. In a skillet, cook ground beef until browned.

5. In a bowl, mix cooked quinoa, cranberries, pecans, feta, cinnamon, salt, and pepper.

6. Fill each squash half with the quinoa mixture and cooked ground beef.

7. Bake for an additional 20 minutes or until squash is tender.

Nutritional Information (per serving):

- Calories: 350

- Protein: 25g

- Carbohydrates: 40g

- Fiber: 8g

- Fat: 15g

- Potassium: 500mg

- Phosphorus: 250mg

9. Lemon Herb Grilled Chicken

Prep Time: 15 minutes

Cooking Time: 15 minutes

Serving Size: 1 chicken breast

Ingredients:

- 1 boneless, skinless chicken breast

- 1 tablespoon olive oil

- 1 tablespoon fresh parsley, chopped

- 1 teaspoon fresh thyme, chopped

- 1 teaspoon fresh rosemary, chopped

- 1 clove garlic, minced

- Zest and juice of 1 lemon

- Salt and pepper to taste

Instructions:

1. Preheat the grill or grill pan over medium-high heat.

2. In a bowl, mix olive oil, parsley, thyme, rosemary, garlic, lemon zest, lemon juice, salt, and pepper.

3. Brush the chicken breast with the herb mixture.

4. Grill for 6-8 minutes per side or until the chicken is cooked through.

5. Let it rest for a few minutes before slicing.

Nutritional Information (per serving):

- Calories: 300

- Protein: 30g

- Carbohydrates: 5g

- Fiber: 1g

- Fat: 15g

- Potassium: 450mg

- Phosphorus: 250mg

10. Shrimp and Broccoli Stir-Fry with Quinoa

Prep Time: 20 minutes

Cooking Time: 15 minutes

Serving Size: 1 stir-fry

Ingredients:

- 6 oz shrimp, peeled and deveined

- 1 cup broccoli florets

- 1/2 cup snap peas

- 1/4 cup carrots, sliced

- 1 cup cooked quinoa

- 2 tablespoons soy sauce (low-sodium)

- 1 tablespoon sesame oil

- 1 clove garlic, minced

- 1 teaspoon ginger, grated

Instructions:

1. In a wok or skillet, heat sesame oil over medium-high heat.

2. Add garlic and ginger, sauté for a minute.

3. Stir in shrimp, broccoli, snap peas, and carrots. Cook until shrimp are pink.

4. Add soy sauce, toss to combine.

5. Serve over cooked quinoa.

Nutritional Information (per serving):

- Calories: 320

- Protein: 25g

- Carbohydrates: 30g

- Fiber: 5g

- Fat: 15g

- Potassium: 400mg

- Phosphorus: 250mg

11. Mediterranean Chickpea Salad

Prep Time: 15 minutes

Cooking Time: 0 minutes

Serving Size: 1 bowl

Ingredients:

- 1 can (15 oz) chickpeas, drained and rinsed

- 1 cucumber, diced

- 1/4 cup cherry tomatoes, halved

- 1/4 cup red onion, finely chopped

- 2 tablespoons Kalamata olives, sliced

- 2 tablespoons feta cheese, crumbled

- 1 tablespoon olive oil

- 1 tablespoon balsamic vinegar

- Fresh oregano for garnish

Instructions:

1. In a bowl, combine chickpeas, cucumber, cherry tomatoes, red onion, olives, and feta cheese.

2. Drizzle with olive oil and balsamic vinegar.

3. Toss gently and garnish with fresh oregano.

4. Enjoy this refreshing and satisfying Mediterranean chickpea salad.

Nutritional Information (per serving):

- Calories: 280

- Protein: 10g

- Carbohydrates: 30g

- Fiber: 8g

- Fat: 15g

- Potassium: 350mg

- Phosphorus: 200mg

12. Turkey and Quinoa Stuffed Peppers

Prep Time: 20 minutes
Cooking Time: 25 minutes
Serving Size: 2 stuffed peppers

Ingredients:

- 1/2 cup cooked quinoa

- 1/2 lb ground turkey

- 2 bell peppers, halved and seeds removed

- 1/4 cup black beans, drained and rinsed

- 1/4 cup corn kernels (fresh or frozen)

- 1/4 cup salsa

- 1/4 cup shredded cheddar cheese

- 1 teaspoon taco seasoning

- Fresh cilantro for garnish

Instructions:

1. Preheat the oven to 375°F (190°C).

2. In a skillet, cook ground turkey until browned.

3. Stir in cooked quinoa, black beans, corn, salsa, and taco seasoning.

4. Fill halved bell peppers with the turkey and quinoa mixture.

5. Top with shredded cheddar cheese and bake for 20-25 minutes.

6. Garnish with fresh cilantro before serving.

Nutritional Information (per serving):

- Calories: 320

- Protein: 25g

- Carbohydrates: 25g

- Fiber: 5g

- Fat: 15g

- Potassium: 400mg

- Phosphorus: 250mg

13. Broccoli and Cheddar Stuffed Baked Potatoes

Prep Time: 15 minutes

Cooking Time: 1 hour

Serving Size: 1 stuffed baked potato

Ingredients:

- 1 large baked potato

- 1 cup broccoli florets, steamed

- 1/4 cup cheddar cheese, shredded

- 2 tablespoons Greek yogurt (unsweetened)

- 1 tablespoon chives, chopped

- Salt and pepper to taste

Instructions:

1. Bake the potato until tender (about 45-60 minutes).

2. Cut the top of the potato and scoop out some of the flesh.

3. Mash the removed potato flesh with Greek yogurt, salt, and pepper.

4. Steam broccoli florets and mix with the mashed potato.

5. Spoon the mixture back into the potato skin.

6. Top with shredded cheddar cheese and chives.

7. Broil for a few minutes until cheese is melted and bubbly.

Nutritional Information (per serving):

- Calories: 280

- Protein: 10g

- Carbohydrates: 40g

- Fiber: 6g

- Fat: 10g

- Potassium: 450mg

- Phosphorus: 250mg

14. Caprese Chicken Skillet

Prep Time: 15 minutes

Cooking Time: 20 minutes

Serving Size: 1 chicken breast

Ingredients:

- 1 boneless, skinless chicken breast

- 1/2 cup cherry tomatoes, halved

- 1/4 cup fresh mozzarella, sliced

- 2 tablespoons balsamic glaze

- Fresh basil leaves for garnish

- Salt and pepper to taste

Instructions:

1. Season chicken breast with salt and pepper.

2. In a skillet, cook chicken over medium heat until no longer pink.

3. Top with cherry tomatoes and mozzarella slices.

4. Cover the skillet until cheese is melted and tomatoes are warmed.

5. Drizzle with balsamic glaze and garnish with fresh basil.

Nutritional Information (per serving):

- Calories: 300

- Protein: 30g

- Carbohydrates: 8g

- Fiber: 2g

- Fat: 15g

- Potassium: 400mg

- Phosphorus: 250mg

15. Cauliflower Fried Rice with Shrimp

Prep Time: 20 minutes

Cooking Time: 15 minutes

Serving Size: 1 serving

Ingredients:

- 6 oz shrimp, peeled and deveined

- 1 cup cauliflower rice

- 1/4 cup carrots, diced

- 1/4 cup peas

- 1/4 cup scallions, chopped

- 1 clove garlic, minced

- 1 tablespoon soy sauce (low-sodium)

- 1 tablespoon sesame oil

- 1 egg, beaten

- Sesame seeds for garnish

Instructions:

1. In a wok or skillet, heat sesame oil over medium-high heat.

2. Add shrimp and cook until pink and opaque.

3. Push shrimp to the side and add minced garlic.

4. Stir in cauliflower rice, carrots, peas, and scallions. Cook until vegetables are tender.

5. Push the mixture to the side and pour the beaten egg into the empty space.

6. Scramble the egg until cooked and mix it into the rice mixture.

7. Add soy sauce, toss well, and garnish with sesame seeds.

Nutritional Information (per serving):

- Calories: 320

- Protein: 25g

- Carbohydrates: 20g

- Fiber: 6g

- Fat: 15g

- Potassium: 400mg

- Phosphorus: 250mg

16. Chicken and Vegetable Kebabs

Prep Time: 20 minutes

Cooking Time: 15 minutes

Serving Size: 2 kebabs

Ingredients:

- 6 oz chicken breast, cut into cubes

- 1/2 cup cherry tomatoes

- 1/2 cup zucchini, sliced

- 1/4 cup red onion, cut into chunks

- 1/4 cup bell peppers, diced

- 1 tablespoon olive oil

- 1 teaspoon Italian seasoning

- Salt and pepper to taste

- Wooden skewers, soaked in water

Instructions:

1. Preheat the grill or grill pan over medium-high heat.

2. In a bowl, combine chicken cubes with olive oil, Italian seasoning, salt, and pepper.

3. Thread chicken, cherry tomatoes, zucchini, red onion, and bell peppers onto skewers.

4. Grill for 10-15 minutes, turning occasionally, until chicken is cooked through.

5. Serve these flavorful kebabs over a bed of quinoa or brown rice.

Nutritional Information (per serving):

- Calories: 300

- Protein: 25g

- Carbohydrates: 20g

- Fiber: 5g

- Fat: 15g

- Potassium: 450mg

- Phosphorus: 250mg

17. Pesto Zucchini Noodles with Grilled Chicken

Prep Time: 15 minutes
Cooking Time: 15 minutes
Serving Size: 1 serving

Ingredients:

- 6 oz chicken breast

- 2 medium zucchinis, spiralized

- 1/4 cup cherry tomatoes, halved

- 2 tablespoons pesto sauce

- 1 tablespoon Parmesan cheese, grated

- Salt and pepper to taste

- Fresh basil leaves for garnish

Instructions:

1. Grill chicken breast until fully cooked.

2. Spiralize zucchinis to create noodles.

3. In a skillet, heat zucchini noodles until just tender.

4. Slice grilled chicken and arrange it on top of the zucchini noodles.

5. Add cherry tomatoes, spoon pesto sauce over the dish, and sprinkle with Parmesan cheese.

6. Garnish with fresh basil leaves before serving.

Nutritional Information (per serving):

- Calories: 320

- Protein: 30g

- Carbohydrates: 10g

- Fiber: 3g

- Fat: 15g

- Potassium: 400mg

- Phosphorus: 250mg

18. Ratatouille with Chicken

Prep Time: 20 minutes

Cooking Time: 25 minutes

Serving Size: 1 serving

Ingredients:

- 6 oz chicken thigh, boneless and skinless

- 1/2 cup eggplant, diced

- 1/2 cup zucchini, diced

- 1/2 cup bell peppers, diced

- 1/2 cup tomatoes, diced

- 1/4 cup onion, finely chopped

- 2 cloves garlic, minced

- 1 tablespoon olive oil

- 1 teaspoon dried thyme

- Salt and pepper to taste

Instructions:

1. Season chicken thigh with salt and pepper.

2. In a skillet, heat olive oil over medium-high heat.

3. Cook chicken until browned on both sides and cooked through.

4. Remove chicken and set aside.

5. In the same skillet, sauté garlic and onion until softened.

6. Add eggplant, zucchini, bell peppers, and tomatoes. Cook until vegetables are tender.

7. Stir in dried thyme and return cooked chicken to the skillet.

8. Simmer for a few minutes until flavors meld together.

Nutritional Information (per serving):

- Calories: 320

- Protein: 25g

- Carbohydrates: 20g

- Fiber: 6g

- Fat: 15g

- Potassium: 450mg

- Phosphorus: 250mg

19. Turkey and Sweet Potato Hash

Prep Time: 20 minutes

Cooking Time: 20 minutes

Serving Size: 1 serving

Ingredients:

- 1/2 lb ground turkey

- 1 medium sweet potato, diced

- 1/4 cup red bell pepper, diced

- 1/4 cup red onion, finely chopped

- 1 clove garlic, minced

- 1 tablespoon olive oil

- 1 teaspoon paprika

- 1/2 teaspoon cumin

- Salt and pepper to taste

- Fresh parsley for garnish

Instructions:

1. In a skillet, heat olive oil over medium heat.

2. Add ground turkey and cook until browned.

3. Stir in sweet potato, red bell pepper, red onion, and garlic.

4. Season with paprika, cumin, salt, and pepper.

5. Cook until sweet potatoes are tender.

6. Garnish with fresh parsley before serving.

Nutritional Information (per serving):

- Calories: 300

- Protein: 20g

- Carbohydrates: 30g

- Fiber: 6g

- Fat: 15g

- Potassium: 400mg

- Phosphorus: 250mg

20. Spinach and Mushroom Stuffed Chicken Breast

Prep Time: 20 minutes

Cooking Time: 25 minutes

Serving Size: 1 stuffed chicken breast

Ingredients:

- 6 oz chicken breast

- 1/2 cup spinach, chopped

- 1/4 cup mushrooms, sliced

- 2 tablespoons feta cheese, crumbled

- 1 clove garlic, minced

- 1 teaspoon olive oil

- Lemon wedges for serving

- Salt and pepper to taste

Instructions:

1. Preheat the oven to 375°F (190°C).

2. In a skillet, sauté mushrooms, garlic, and spinach in olive oil until wilted.

3. Butterfly the chicken breast and stuff with sautéed spinach, mushrooms, and feta.

4. Season with salt and pepper, then secure with toothpicks.

5. Bake for 25 minutes or until chicken is cooked through.

6. Serve with lemon wedges for a burst of freshness.

Nutritional Information (per serving):

- Calories: 280

- Protein: 30g

- Carbohydrates: 5g

- Fiber: 2g

- Fat: 15g

- Potassium: 400mg

- Phosphorus: 250mg

DESSERT RECIPES

1. Berry Chia Seed Pudding

Prep Time: 10 minutes

Cooking Time: 0 minutes

Serving Size: 1 pudding cup

Ingredients:

- 2 tablespoons chia seeds

- 1/2 cup unsweetened almond milk

- 1/4 cup mixed berries (blueberries, raspberries, strawberries)

- 1 teaspoon vanilla extract

- 1/2 tablespoon honey or a sugar substitute

Instructions:

1. In a bowl, mix chia seeds, almond milk, vanilla extract, and honey.

2. Let it sit in the refrigerator for at least 2 hours or overnight.

3. Before serving, layer the chia pudding with mixed berries.

4. Enjoy this delightful and fiber-rich dessert.

Nutritional Information (per serving):

- Calories: 150

- Protein: 4g

- Carbohydrates: 20g

- Fiber: 8g

- Fat: 6g

- Potassium: 180mg

- Phosphorus: 100mg

2. Avocado Chocolate Mousse

Prep Time: 15 minutes
Cooking Time: 0 minutes
Serving Size: 1/2 cup

Ingredients:

- 1 ripe avocado

- 2 tablespoons unsweetened cocoa powder

- 2 tablespoons almond milk

- 1/4 cup sugar-free sweetener

- 1 teaspoon vanilla extract

- Pinch of salt

Instructions:

1. Blend avocado, cocoa powder, almond milk, sweetener, vanilla extract, and a pinch of salt until smooth.

2. Refrigerate for at least 1 hour before serving.

3. Serve this creamy and rich chocolate mousse in small portions.

Nutritional Information (per serving):

- Calories: 120

- Protein: 2g

- Carbohydrates: 10g

- Fiber: 6g

- Fat: 9g

- Potassium: 250mg

- Phosphorus: 60mg

3. Greek Yogurt Parfait with Nuts and Berries

Prep Time: 10 minutes

Cooking Time: 0 minutes

Serving Size: 1 parfait

Ingredients:

- 1/2 cup Greek yogurt (unsweetened)

- 1/4 cup mixed berries (strawberries, blueberries)

- 1 tablespoon chopped nuts (almonds, walnuts)

- 1/2 tablespoon honey or a sugar substitute

Instructions:

1. In a glass, layer Greek yogurt with mixed berries and chopped nuts.

2. Drizzle honey or a sugar substitute over the top.

3. Create multiple layers for a visually appealing parfait.

4. Indulge in this protein-packed and satisfying dessert.

Nutritional Information (per serving):

- Calories: 180

- Protein: 10g

- Carbohydrates: 15g

- Fiber: 3g

- Fat: 9g

- Potassium: 200mg

- Phosphorus: 100mg

4. Baked Apple with Cinnamon and Walnuts

Prep Time: 15 minutes

Cooking Time: 30 minutes

Serving Size: 1 baked apple

Ingredients:

- 1 medium-sized apple, cored

- 1/2 tablespoon lemon juice

- 1/2 teaspoon ground cinnamon

- 1 tablespoon chopped walnuts

- 1/2 tablespoon honey or a sugar substitute

Instructions:

1. Preheat the oven to 375°F (190°C).

2. Place the cored apple in a baking dish.

3. Drizzle lemon juice over the apple.

4. Sprinkle with cinnamon and stuff with chopped walnuts.

5. Bake for 30 minutes or until the apple is tender.

6. Drizzle honey or a sugar substitute before serving.

Nutritional Information (per serving):

- Calories: 150

- Protein: 2g

- Carbohydrates: 25g

- Fiber: 5g

- Fat: 6g

- Potassium: 180mg

- Phosphorus: 40mg

5. Coconut Chia Seed Pudding with Mango

Prep Time: 10 minutes

Cooking Time: 0 minutes

Serving Size: 1 pudding cup

Ingredients:

- 2 tablespoons chia seeds

- 1/2 cup coconut milk (unsweetened)

- 1/4 cup diced mango

- 1/2 tablespoon agave syrup or a sugar substitute

- 1/2 tablespoon shredded coconut (unsweetened)

Instructions:

1. Mix chia seeds and coconut milk in a bowl.

2. Let it sit in the refrigerator for at least 2 hours or overnight.

3. Layer with diced mango and top with shredded coconut.

4. Drizzle agave syrup or a sugar substitute for sweetness.

Nutritional Information (per serving):

- Calories: 180

- Protein: 4g

- Carbohydrates: 15g

- Fiber: 7g

- Fat: 12g

- Potassium: 200mg

- Phosphorus: 90mg

6. Pumpkin Spice Chia Pudding

Prep Time: 10 minutes
Cooking Time: 0 minutes
Serving Size: 1 pudding cup

Ingredients:

- 2 tablespoons chia seeds

- 1/2 cup unsweetened almond milk

- 2 tablespoons canned pumpkin puree

- 1/2 teaspoon pumpkin spice

- 1/2 tablespoon maple syrup or a sugar substitute

- 1 tablespoon chopped pecans

Instructions:

1. Combine chia seeds, almond milk, pumpkin puree, pumpkin spice, and maple syrup in a bowl.

2. Refrigerate for at least 2 hours or overnight.

3. Top with chopped pecans before serving.

4. Savor the fall flavors in this nutritious pudding.

Nutritional Information (per serving):

- Calories: 160

- Protein: 4g

- Carbohydrates: 15g

- Fiber: 8g

- Fat: 10g

- Potassium: 180mg

- Phosphorus: 80mg

7. Almond Flour Banana Bread

Prep Time: 15 minutes

Cooking Time: 45 minutes

Serving Size: 1 slice

Ingredients:

- 1 cup almond flour

- 2 ripe bananas, mashed

- 2 eggs

- 1/4 cup coconut oil, melted

- 1 teaspoon vanilla extract

- 1/2 teaspoon baking soda

- Pinch of salt

- 1/4 cup chopped almonds for topping

Instructions:

1. Preheat the oven to 350°F (175°C).

2. In a bowl, mix almond flour, mashed bananas, eggs, melted coconut oil, vanilla extract, baking soda, and salt.

3. Pour the batter into a greased loaf pan.

4. Sprinkle chopped almonds on top.

5. Bake for 45 minutes or until a toothpick comes out clean.

Nutritional Information (per serving):

- Calories: 200

- Protein: 6g

- Carbohydrates: 15g

- Fiber: 3g

- Fat: 15g

- Potassium: 220mg

- Phosphorus: 60mg

8. Raspberry Almond Flour Muffins

Prep Time: 15 minutes
Cooking Time: 20 minutes
Serving Size: 1 muffin

Ingredients:

- 1 cup almond flour

- 1/2 cup raspberries

- 2 eggs

- 1/4 cup almond milk (unsweetened)

- 2 tablespoons coconut oil, melted

- 1/4 cup sugar-free sweetener

- 1/2 teaspoon baking powder

- 1/2 teaspoon almond extract

Instructions:

1. Preheat the oven to 350°F (175°C).

2. In a bowl, mix almond flour, raspberries, eggs, almond milk, melted coconut oil, sweetener, baking powder, and almond extract.

3. Spoon the batter into muffin cups.

4. Bake for 20 minutes or until golden brown.

Nutritional Information (per serving):

- Calories: 180

- Protein: 6g

- Carbohydrates: 10g

- Fiber: 3g

- Fat: 14g

- Potassium: 140mg

- Phosphorus: 50mg

9. Cinnamon Apple Walnut Oatmeal Bake

Prep Time: 15 minutes

Cooking Time: 30 minutes

Serving Size: 1 square

Ingredients:

- 1 cup rolled oats

- 1/2 cup unsweetened applesauce

- 1/4 cup chopped walnuts

- 1/4 cup diced apples

- 2 tablespoons maple syrup or a sugar substitute

- 1 teaspoon cinnamon

- 1/2 teaspoon baking powder

- Pinch of salt

Instructions:

1. Preheat the oven to 350°F (175°C).

2. In a bowl, combine rolled oats, applesauce, chopped walnuts, diced apples, maple syrup, cinnamon, baking powder, and salt.

3. Spread the mixture evenly in a greased baking dish.

4. Bake for 30 minutes or until golden brown.

5. Cut into squares and serve warm.

Nutritional Information (per serving):

- Calories: 220

- Protein: 5g

- Carbohydrates: 30g

- Fiber: 5g

- Fat: 9g

- Potassium: 180mg

- Phosphorus: 100mg

10. Chocolate Avocado Mousse with Berries

Prep Time: 15 minutes
Cooking Time: 0 minutes
Serving Size: 1/2 cup

Ingredients:

- 1 ripe avocado

- 2 tablespoons unsweetened cocoa powder

- 2 tablespoons almond milk

- 1/4 cup mixed berries (strawberries, blueberries)

- 1/2 tablespoon honey or a sugar substitute

- Mint leaves for garnish

Instructions:

1. Blend avocado, cocoa powder, almond milk, and honey until smooth.

2. Refrigerate for at least 1 hour.

3. Serve topped with mixed berries and garnish with mint leaves.

4. Enjoy this decadent and healthy chocolate mousse.

Nutritional Information (per serving):

- Calories: 160

- Protein: 3g

- Carbohydrates: 15g

- Fiber: 7g

- Fat: 11g

- Potassium: 270mg

- Phosphorus: 60mg

35-DAY MEAL PLAN

Day 1:

- **Breakfast:** Spinach and Feta Omelette

- **Lunch:** Lentil and Vegetable Soup

- **Dinner:** Baked Lemon Herb Salmon

- **Snack:** Nuts and Seeds Energy Bites

- **Dessert:** Berry Chia Seed Pudding

Day 2:

- **Breakfast:** Overnight Chia Seed Pudding with Berries

- **Lunch:** Turkey and Avocado Wrap

- **Dinner:** Chickpea and Spinach Curry

- **Snack:** Greek Yogurt with Berries and Almonds

- **Dessert:** Avocado Chocolate Mousse

Day 3:

- **Breakfast:** Quinoa Breakfast Bowl with Fruit

- **Lunch:** Quinoa and Black Bean Bowl

- **Dinner:** Chicken Parmesan with Zucchini Noodles

- **Snack:** Hummus and Veggie Sticks

163

- **Dessert:** Greek Yogurt Parfait with Nuts and Berries

Day 4:

- **Breakfast:** Sweet Potato and Turkey Breakfast Hash

- **Lunch:** Mediterranean Chickpea Salad

- **Dinner:** Teriyaki Tofu Stir-Fry

- **Snack:** Cottage Cheese with Pineapple

- **Dessert:** Baked Apple with Cinnamon and Walnuts

Day 5:

- **Breakfast:** Greek Yogurt Parfait with Granola

- **Lunch:** Turkey and Quinoa Stuffed Peppers

- **Dinner:** Quinoa-Stuffed Bell Peppers

- **Snack:** Avocado and Tomato Salsa

- **Dessert:** Coconut Chia Seed Pudding with Mango

Day 6:

- **Breakfast:** Blueberry Almond Flour Pancakes

- **Lunch:** Broccoli and Cheddar Stuffed Baked Potatoes

- **Dinner:** Shrimp and Vegetable Stir-Fry with Quinoa

- **Snack:** Apple Slices with Almond Butter

- **Dessert:** Pumpkin Spice Chia Pudding

Day 7:

- **Breakfast:** Veggie and Cheese Breakfast Burrito

- **Lunch:** Caprese Chicken Skillet

- **Dinner:** Mediterranean Chicken Skewers

- **Snack:** Edamame Guacamole

- **Dessert:** Almond Flour Banana Bread

Day 8:

- **Breakfast:** Smoked Salmon and Cream Cheese Bagel

- **Lunch:** Cauliflower Fried Rice with Shrimp

- **Dinner:** Black Bean and Vegetable Quesadilla

- **Snack:** Cucumber and Tuna Bites

- **Dessert:** Raspberry Almond Flour Muffins

Day 9:

- **Breakfast:** Banana Walnut Oatmeal

- **Lunch:** Chicken and Vegetable Kebabs

- **Dinner:** Creamy Garlic Parmesan Spaghetti Squash

- **Snack:** Roasted Chickpeas

- **Dessert:** Cinnamon Apple Walnut Oatmeal Bake

Day 10:

- **Breakfast:** Zucchini and Mushroom Frittata

- **Lunch:** Pesto Zucchini Noodles with Grilled Chicken

- **Dinner:** Grilled Veggie and Hummus Wrap

- **Snack:** Dark Chocolate-Dipped Strawberries

- **Dessert:** Chocolate Avocado Mousse with Berries

Day 11:

- **Breakfast:** Peanut Butter Banana Smoothie Bowl

- **Lunch:** Ratatouille with Chicken

- **Dinner:** Sesame Ginger Tofu with Brown Rice

- **Snack:** Greek Yogurt with Berries and Almonds

- **Dessert:** Berry Chia Seed Pudding

Day 12:

- **Breakfast:** Egg and Veggie Breakfast Wrap

- **Lunch:** Turkey and Sweet Potato Hash

- **Dinner:** Lemon Herb Chicken and Asparagus

- **Snack:** Hummus and Veggie Sticks

- **Dessert:** Avocado Chocolate Mousse

Day 13:

- **Breakfast:** Mango Coconut Chia Pudding

- **Lunch:** Spinach and Mushroom Stuffed Chicken Breast

- **Dinner:** Quinoa and Vegetable Stir-Fry

- **Snack:** Cottage Cheese with Pineapple

- **Dessert:** Greek Yogurt Parfait with Nuts and Berries

Day 14:

- **Breakfast:** Whole Grain Toast with Avocado and Poached Egg

- **Lunch:** Chickpea and Spinach Curry

- **Dinner:** Quinoa and Black Bean Stuffed Acorn Squash

- **Snack:** Apple Slices with Almond Butter

- **Dessert:** Baked Apple with Cinnamon and Walnuts

Day 15:

- **Breakfast:** Strawberry Protein Smoothie

- **Lunch:** Greek Salad with Grilled Shrimp

- **Dinner:** Sweet Potato and Chickpea Curry

- **Snack:** Nuts and Seeds Energy Bites

- **Dessert:** Coconut Chia Seed Pudding with Mango

Day 16:

- **Breakfast:** Oat Bran Porridge with Mixed Berries

- **Lunch:** Quinoa and Vegetable Stir-Fry

- **Dinner:** Garlic Shrimp and Broccoli Stir-Fry

- **Snack:** Avocado and Tomato Salsa

- **Dessert:** Pumpkin Spice Chia Pudding

Day 17:

- **Breakfast:** Veggie and Sausage Breakfast Casserole

- **Lunch:** Mediterranean Tuna Salad

- **Dinner:** Mediterranean Quinoa Salad with Grilled Vegetables

- **Snack:** Cucumber and Tuna Bites

- **Dessert:** Almond Flour Banana Bread

Day 18:

- **Breakfast:** Green Tea Smoothie with Spinach and Pineapple

- **Lunch:** Sweet Potato and Black Bean Quesadilla

- **Dinner:** Beef and Broccoli Stir-Fry

- **Snack:** Roasted Chickpeas

- **Dessert:** Raspberry Almond Flour Muffins

Day 19:

- **Breakfast:** Breakfast Quinoa with Almond Milk and Berries

- **Lunch:** Salmon and Asparagus Foil Packets

- **Dinner:** Grilled Veggie and Hummus Wrap

- **Snack:** Dark Chocolate-Dipped Strawberries

- **Dessert:** Chocolate Avocado Mousse with Berries

Day 20:

- **Breakfast:** Sweet Potato and Turkey Breakfast Hash

- **Lunch:** Broccoli and Cheddar Stuffed Baked Potatoes

- **Dinner:** Shrimp and Vegetable Stir-Fry with Quinoa

- **Snack:** Apple Slices with Almond Butter

- **Dessert:** Pumpkin Spice Chia Pudding

Day 21:

- **Breakfast:** Greek Yogurt Parfait with Granola

- **Lunch:** Caprese Chicken Skillet

- **Dinner:** Mediterranean Chicken Skewers

- **Snack:** Edamame Guacamole

- **Dessert:** Almond Flour Banana Bread

Day 22:

- **Breakfast:** Smoked Salmon and Cream Cheese Bagel

- **Lunch:** Cauliflower Fried Rice with Shrimp

- **Dinner:** Black Bean and Vegetable Quesadilla

- **Snack:** Cucumber and Tuna Bites

- **Dessert:** Raspberry Almond Flour Muffins

Day 23:

- **Breakfast:** Banana Walnut Oatmeal

- **Lunch:** Chicken and Vegetable Kebabs

- **Dinner:** Creamy Garlic Parmesan Spaghetti Squash

- **Snack:** Roasted Chickpeas

- **Dessert:** Cinnamon Apple Walnut Oatmeal Bake

Day 24:

- **Breakfast:** Zucchini and Mushroom Frittata

- **Lunch:** Pesto Zucchini Noodles with Grilled Chicken

- **Dinner:** Grilled Veggie and Hummus Wrap

- **Snack:** Dark Chocolate-Dipped Strawberries

- **Dessert:** Chocolate Avocado Mousse with Berries

Day 25:

- **Breakfast:** Peanut Butter Banana Smoothie Bowl

- **Lunch:** Ratatouille with Chicken

- **Dinner:** Sesame Ginger Tofu with Brown Rice

- **Snack:** Greek Yogurt with Berries and Almonds

- **Dessert:** Berry Chia Seed Pudding

Day 26:

- **Breakfast:** Egg and Veggie Breakfast Wrap

- **Lunch:** Turkey and Sweet Potato Hash

- **Dinner:** Lemon Herb Chicken and Asparagus

- **Snack:** Hummus and Veggie Sticks

- **Dessert:** Avocado Chocolate Mousse

Day 27:

- **Breakfast:** Mango Coconut Chia Pudding

- **Lunch:** Spinach and Mushroom Stuffed Chicken Breast

- **Dinner:** Quinoa and Vegetable Stir-Fry

- **Snack:** Cottage Cheese with Pineapple

- **Dessert:** Greek Yogurt Parfait with Nuts and Berries

Day 28:

- **Breakfast:** Whole Grain Toast with Avocado and Poached Egg

- **Lunch:** Chickpea and Spinach Curry

- **Dinner:** Quinoa and Black Bean Stuffed Acorn Squash

- **Snack:** Apple Slices with Almond Butter

- **Dessert:** Baked Apple with Cinnamon and Walnuts

Day 29:

- **Breakfast:** Strawberry Protein Smoothie

- **Lunch:** Greek Salad with Grilled Shrimp

- **Dinner:** Sweet Potato and Chickpea Curry

- **Snack:** Nuts and Seeds Energy Bites

- **Dessert:** Coconut Chia Seed Pudding with Mango

Day 30:

- **Breakfast:** Oat Bran Porridge with Mixed Berries

- **Lunch:** Quinoa and Vegetable Stir-Fry

- **Dinner:** Garlic Shrimp and Broccoli Stir-Fry

- **Snack:** Avocado and Tomato Salsa

- **Dessert:** Pumpkin Spice Chia Pudding

Day 31:

- **Breakfast:** Veggie and Sausage Breakfast Casserole

- **Lunch:** Mediterranean Tuna Salad

- **Dinner:** Mediterranean Quinoa Salad with Grilled Vegetables

- **Snack:** Cucumber and Tuna Bites

- **Dessert:** Almond Flour Banana Bread

Day 32:

- **Breakfast:** Green Tea Smoothie with Spinach and Pineapple

- **Lunch:** Sweet Potato and Black Bean Quesadilla

- **Dinner:** Beef and Broccoli Stir-Fry

- **Snack:** Roasted Chickpeas

- **Dessert:** Raspberry Almond Flour Muffins

Day 33:

- **Breakfast:** Breakfast Quinoa with Almond Milk and Berries

- **Lunch:** Salmon and Asparagus Foil Packets

- **Dinner:** Grilled Veggie and Hummus Wrap

- **Snack:** Dark Chocolate-Dipped Strawberries

- **Dessert:** Chocolate Avocado Mousse with Berries

Day 34:

- **Breakfast:** Sweet Potato and Turkey Breakfast Hash

- **Lunch:** Broccoli and Cheddar Stuffed Baked Potatoes

- **Dinner:** Shrimp and Vegetable Stir-Fry with Quinoa

- **Snack:** Apple Slices with Almond Butter

- **Dessert:** Pumpkin Spice Chia Pudding

Day 35:

- **Breakfast:** Greek Yogurt Parfait with Granola

- **Lunch:** Caprese Chicken Skillet

- **Dinner:** Mediterranean Chicken Skewers

- **Snack:** Edamame Guacamole

- **Dessert:** Almond Flour Banana Bread

LIFESTYLE TIPS FOR MANAGING CKD AND DIABETES

Living with both Chronic Kidney Disease (CKD) Stage 3 and Type 2 Diabetes requires a holistic approach to health and well-being. Adopting a mindful lifestyle can significantly contribute to the effective management of these conditions. In this section, we'll explore three key lifestyle tips that can make a substantial difference in promoting overall health and mitigating the impact of CKD and Diabetes.

Incorporating Physical Activity

Physical activity plays a pivotal role in the management of CKD and Diabetes. While it may seem counterintuitive to engage in exercise when dealing with chronic health conditions, the right type and amount of physical activity can offer numerous benefits. Regular exercise contributes to improved blood circulation, weight management, and enhanced insulin sensitivity, which are crucial for individuals with Type 2 Diabetes.

For those with CKD Stage 3, it's important to tailor the exercise routine to individual capabilities and adhere to any restrictions provided by healthcare professionals. Low-impact exercises such as walking, swimming, and cycling can be excellent choices. These activities not only promote cardiovascular health but also reduce the risk of complications associated with diabetes, such as cardiovascular disease.

Strength training is another valuable component of an exercise regimen. It helps maintain muscle mass, aids in weight management, and improves overall metabolic function. However, it's essential to consult with healthcare providers before starting any new exercise program to ensure that it aligns with individual health needs.

Moreover, integrating physical activity into daily life need not be overly strenuous. Simple lifestyle modifications, such as taking short walks after meals, using stairs instead of elevators, and incorporating stretching routines, can contribute significantly to improved health outcomes.

Stress Management Techniques

Stress, whether physical or emotional, can have profound effects on both diabetes and CKD. Chronic stress can elevate blood sugar levels and exacerbate kidney-related issues. Therefore, incorporating stress management techniques is crucial for individuals navigating the complex terrain of CKD Stage 3 and Type 2 Diabetes.

Mindfulness practices, such as meditation and deep breathing exercises, are effective tools for stress reduction. These techniques promote relaxation, alleviate anxiety, and enhance overall emotional well-being. Engaging in activities that bring joy and relaxation, such as reading, listening to music, or spending time in nature, can also contribute to stress reduction.

Building a robust support system is an often overlooked but invaluable aspect of stress management. Sharing concerns, experiences, and emotions with friends, family, or support groups can provide emotional relief and foster a sense of connection. It's essential to recognize that managing chronic health conditions can be challenging, and seeking support is a sign of strength, not weakness.

In some cases, professional counseling or therapy may be beneficial for addressing specific stressors and developing coping mechanisms. Healthcare providers can guide individuals to resources that offer specialized support for managing the emotional aspects of living with CKD and Diabetes.

Regular Monitoring of Blood Sugar and Kidney Function

Regular monitoring is the cornerstone of effective management for both CKD Stage 3 and Type 2 Diabetes. Keeping a vigilant eye on blood sugar levels and kidney function allows for timely adjustments to treatment plans and helps prevent complications.

For individuals with diabetes, continuous glucose monitoring or regular self-monitoring of blood glucose levels is essential. This empowers individuals to make informed decisions about dietary choices, medication adjustments, and overall lifestyle modifications. Regular monitoring helps maintain glycemic control, reducing the risk of hyperglycemia and hypoglycemia, both of which can have adverse effects on kidney function.

Kidney function monitoring involves regular check-ups and laboratory tests, including estimated glomerular filtration rate (eGFR) and urinary albumin tests. These assessments provide insights into the health of the kidneys and help healthcare providers identify any deterioration in function early on.

Adhering to prescribed medications and treatment plans is crucial for maintaining stable blood sugar levels and supporting kidney health. Regular communication with healthcare providers ensures that any changes in health status or medication requirements are promptly addressed.

CONCLUSION

As we reach the end of the "CKD Stage 3 and Diabetes Type 2 Cookbook for Beginners," it's not just the closing of a book but the beginning of a journey towards a healthier, more flavorful life. The culinary adventure we embarked on together wasn't just about recipes; it was about understanding the art of nourishing our bodies, especially when dealing with the intricate dance of CKD Stage 3 and Type 2 Diabetes.

In these pages, we explored the delicate balance of flavors, textures, and nutritional goodness tailored to the unique needs of those managing CKD and Diabetes. From the vibrant hues of nutrient-rich vegetables to the subtle symphony of herbs and spices, each recipe was a step towards reclaiming control over our health, one delicious bite at a time.

The heart of this cookbook lies not just in the ingredients listed or the meticulous instructions; it's in the stories shared, the kitchen mishaps laughed off, and the victories celebrated. It's about creating meals that resonate with more than just our taste buds – they resonate with our well-being, our vitality, and our journey towards a more vibrant life.

Through the diverse array of breakfasts, lunches, dinners, snacks, and desserts, we've crafted a repertoire of culinary creations that cater to the specific needs of CKD Stage 3 and Type 2 Diabetes. But beyond the tangible recipes, the essence lies in the empowerment to make informed choices about what we put on our plates.

Cooking for health doesn't mean sacrificing flavor or variety. Instead, it's an invitation to explore the richness of diverse ingredients and savor the joy that comes from nurturing our bodies. Whether it's the simplicity of a nourishing smoothie or the complexity of a well-balanced dinner, each dish carries a message – a message of self-care, resilience, and the belief that we can thrive despite the challenges we face.

As we bid adieu to the last page, let's not see it as a farewell but as a 'see you soon.' The kitchen remains our canvas, and the ingredients are our palette. The lessons learned from these recipes go beyond the culinary realm – they extend to the choices we make for our health every day.

Remember, the "Ckd Stage 3 and Diabetes Type 2 Cookbook for Beginners" isn't just a compilation of recipes; it's a companion in your health journey. It's a reminder that cooking is an expression of self-love and a powerful tool in managing health conditions. May these recipes continue to grace your tables, bringing not just nourishment but a celebration of the vitality within you.

Made in the USA
Las Vegas, NV
21 November 2024

12307152R00105